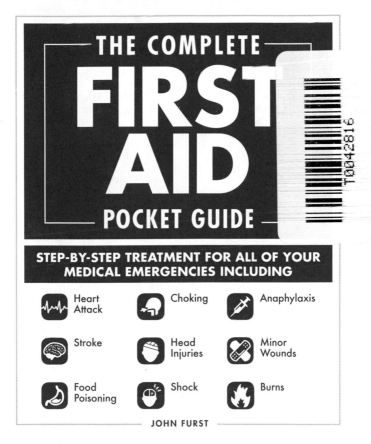

THE COMPLETE
FIRST
AID
POCKET GUIDE

STEP-BY-STEP TREATMENT FOR ALL OF YOUR MEDICAL EMERGENCIES INCLUDING

Heart Attack

Choking

Anaphylaxis

Stroke

Head Injuries

Minor Wounds

Food Poisoning

Shock

Burns

JOHN FURST

Adams Media
New York London Toronto Sydney New Delhi

Aadamsmedia

Adams Media
An Imprint of Simon & Schuster, LLC
100 Technology Center Drive
Stoughton, Massachusetts 02072

First Adams Media trade paperback edition
November 2018

ADAMS MEDIA and colophon are trademarks
of Simon & Schuster.

For information about special discounts for bulk
purchases, please contact Simon & Schuster
Special Sales at 1-866-506-1949 or
business@simonandschuster.com.

The Simon & Schuster Speakers Bureau can bring
authors to your live event. For more information
or to book an event contact the Simon & Schuster
Speakers Bureau at 1-866-248-3049 or visit our
website at www.simonspeakers.com.

Interior design by Michelle Kelly
Interior images by Dave Forbes
Technical review by Robin Miller, MD, MHS

Manufactured in the United States of America

10 9

Library of Congress Cataloging-in-Publication
Data
Furst, John, author.
The complete first aid pocket guide / John Furst.
Avon, Massachusetts: Adams Media, 2018.
Includes index.
LCCN 2018024004 (print) |
LCCN 2018025707 (ebook) | ISBN
9781507208885 (pb) | ISBN 9781507208892
(ebook)
Subjects: LCSH: First aid in illness and
injury--Handbooks, manuals, etc. | Medical
emergencies--Handbooks, manuals, etc. |
BISAC: HEALTH & FITNESS / First Aid. |
MEDICAL / Emergency Medicine.
Classification: LCC RC86.8 (ebook) | LCC RC86.8
.F87 2018 (print) | DDC 616.02/52--dc23
LC record available at https://lccn.loc
.gov/2018024004

ISBN 978-1-5072-0888-5
ISBN 978-1-5072-0889-2 (ebook)

Contents

Chapter 3:
Lifesaving Skills / 45

Chapter 4:
Minor Injuries and Conditions / 77

Chapter 5:
Common Illnesses / 107

Chapter 6:
Traumatic Injuries / 125

Chapter 7:
Medical Emergencies / 163

Chapter 8:
Pediatric Emergencies and Illnesses / 205

Chapter 9:
Environmental Conditions / 239

Chapter 10:
Bites and Stings / 257

Introduction:
What Is First Aid?

Chances are good that at some point in your life, you'll need to provide first aid to someone who's ill or injured. First aid is the initial care you give to a victim before the arrival of professional medical help, and it can make an important difference in the outcome of an illness or accident—sometimes literally the difference between life and death.

In *The Complete First Aid Pocket Guide* you'll be shown what to do in the case of a victim who is unresponsive, how to treat wounds and broken bones, and what to do if someone is having a heart attack or stroke. The book explains how to treat hypothermia or heatstroke and how to protect against sunburn. You'll also be shown the proper way to administer cardiopulmonary resuscitation (CPR), a lifesaving skill most people associate with first aid.

This book will show you how to make a quick assessment of a first aid situation and take measures to stabilize the victim.

In any emergency, in addition to the technical help you can offer, an important role is to provide comfort and reassurance and to coordinate calling for professional assistance. Don't underestimate the power of a calm, reassuring presence to a victim suffering an emergency.

The book is structured to be a quick reference guide. Each section gives a basic introduction to the condition or emergency situation, then describes the common signs and symptoms and first aid treatment. The list of signs and symptoms focuses on the key features of the condition so you can recognize it and offer the appropriate initial first aid treatment. Illustrations throughout the book provide handy reference guides for you to follow.

First aid does not have to be overly complicated or require in-depth medical knowledge. You never know when you might encounter a first aid emergency, so be prepared!

Always Seek Medical Advice

Please remember that this book does not replace professional medical advice from a trained medical practitioner. You must always seek medical assistance for a victim from a suitably qualified professional without delay. Nor does the book replace a hands-on first aid and CPR course from an accredited first aid training provider. After buying this book, consider signing up for a first aid and CPR class in your area so you can have hands-on practice of essential first aid skills. Many local fire departments offer free CPR training sessions for the general public. In addition, the Stop the Bleed campaign (www.bleedingcontrol.org) runs free training classes that teach you how to respond to an injured victim who is bleeding badly. If you want more in-depth training, then the Red Cross runs a wide range of first aid and CPR classes. You can find your closest Red Cross class at www.redcross.org/take-a-class. Your employer may also provide accredited first aid training classes to enable you to take on the role of a first-aider in the workplace.

If you have young children or are expecting a child, it's important to sign up for a local pediatric first aid class. Children and babies are at greater risk of developing serious medical conditions such as asthma and meningitis. In addition, accidental death (for example, from choking) remains a leading cause of death among young children. You can prepare yourself for caring for your child by learning how to act in an emergency situation and give your child the best care possible.

Chapter One
WHAT FIRST AID IS AND ISN'T

FIRST AID is all about providing initial lifesaving care before the arrival of professional help. In first aid, your main aim is to preserve the life of the victim until she can be treated by EMS or another medical professional. A first-aider is someone who has undertaken formal first aid training but is not a professionally trained emergency worker such as a paramedic, firefighter, or first responder. Reading this book is a good way to learn about basic first aid techniques but does not replace attending an authorized and accredited first aid class. In a first aid situation, you are not expected to act as a paramedic or doctor and perform advanced medical procedures. Don't believe everything you watch in films; you won't be performing any open-heart surgery at the roadside or diagnosing complex medical problems! Instead, you should focus on basic lifesaving interventions to keep the victim alive and stable until EMS arrives to take over.

Examples of things you can do in first aid to save the life of your victim include:

- Opening an unconscious victim's airway and placing him in the recovery position (Chapter 3)
- Performing cardiopulmonary resuscitation (CPR) and using an automated external defibrillator (Chapter 3)
- Stopping life-threatening bleeding and recognizing when a victim is going into shock (Chapter 6)
- Recognizing the signs of a life-threatening medical condition, such as meningitis or a heart attack, and calling for EMS early (Chapter 7)
- Cooling a victim who has gone into life-threatening heatstroke (Chapter 9)

After preserving life, your next aim is to prevent the worsening of the victim's condition. You may not be able to fix the underlying problem affecting the victim. For example, you cannot stop a seizure, but you can prevent worsening of the situation by ensuring the victim's airway is open and protected after the seizure has resolved. In the case of a suspected neck or back injury, you cannot fix the underlying damage to the spine, but you can prevent the injury from worsening by keeping the victim as still as possible until EMS arrives to take over care.

Finally, your last aim is to promote recovery from the injury or illness. The action you take in the first few minutes of an emergency situation can have a significant impact on the victim's long-term recovery. For example, quickly cooling a major burn will slow down the burning process and reduce the risk of permanent scarring. Another example is performing early effective CPR on a victim of sudden cardiac arrest when the heart has stopped beating properly. Studies have shown that early CPR is associated with a much better chance of the victim making a full recovery from cardiac arrest.

The Overall Aims of First Aid

You can remember your overall aims in first aid by using the three Ps. They are:

- **P**reserve the life of the victim
- **P**revent worsening of the situation
- **P**romote recovery from the injury or illness

You may recognize the signs of a life-threatening medical condition such as a stroke (brain attack) or meningitis. These victims require early advanced medical care to have the best chance of recovery. Although you won't be expected to perform this advanced medical care, you can really make a difference by being confident in recognizing the warning signs of these serious conditions and calling for help early.

Your Role in a First Aid Situation

In an emergency, the most obvious role you have is to provide the appropriate first aid for the victim's injury or medical condition. However, you have other roles to carry out in order to manage the situation effectively and provide the best care possible to the victim. Let's take a closer look at some of these responsibilities of a first-aider.

When an incident occurs, you may be expected to take charge of the situation before the arrival of professional help. The following section, Managing an Incident, will walk you through this process. You may have to delegate tasks (for example, calling for help) to other bystanders. You'll need to assume this leadership role during an emergency and take control of the situation prior to emergency responders arriving. People will look to you for guidance, and you may be the only person around with an understanding of first aid. Try to keep calm and provide clear instructions to bystanders. If there are multiple victims, you can instruct bystanders to perform basic first aid tasks such as applying pressure to a bleeding wound.

You also need to ensure that the appropriate professional help has been summoned. Normally, this will involve dialing 911 and speaking to an emergency operator (see Calling Emergency Services later in this chapter). However, if you are in a remote location and unable to telephone for help, you may need to delegate someone to go and seek assistance. It is vital that you ensure emergency services are called early so the victim receives timely medical treatment.

When providing first aid to a victim or victims, recording your actions and any important information is important to enable an effective handover to EMS when they arrive. You may be expected to fill out specific first aid paperwork depending on the location and severity of the incident. You should take this aspect seriously, although it can seem unimportant when in the middle of a stressful emergency situation. The accurate handover of information to EMS is critical to ensure the victim receives safe ongoing medical care.

You also have a responsibility to your health and well-being. Your safety is paramount when dealing with an emergency situation. Don't put yourself in danger; you will be unable to help the victim if you are also injured. It can seem unnatural, but you are always the most important person in any situation!

Roles and Responsibilities in First Aid

- Ensure your safety and the safety of bystanders.
- Manage an incident properly and control the situation.
- Call for appropriate emergency services.
- Delegate tasks to bystanders as required.
- Provide appropriate first aid to victims.
- Document your findings and actions.
- Provide an accurate handover to EMS.

Managing an Incident

When an emergency situation occurs, there is often panic among bystanders and victims. In this section, we will look at how to manage an incident and take control of an emergency situation before the arrival of professional help.

The priority in managing any incident is to ensure the scene is safe for you and others to approach. You should conduct a quick assessment of any hazards that might be present. A hazard is anything with the potential to cause harm (see sidebar, Potential Hazards in a First Aid Situation). Make sure you conduct this assessment before rushing in to provide aid to a victim. Otherwise, you run the risk of becoming an additional victim, making you unable to render any aid.

If you identify a hazard, then you should take steps to reduce the risk of harm to yourself, bystanders, and the victim. For example, move the victim away from the hazard if possible. If you decide the scene is too dangerous to approach, then stay clear and immediately contact emergency services.

Potential Hazards in a First Aid Situation

- Fast-moving traffic
- Slip and trip hazards
- Extremes of temperature
- Deep or fast-moving water
- Electrical appliances or exposed wires
- The victim, if she or he is under the influence of alcohol or recreational drugs
- Other people (for example, during an altercation)
- Poisons (for example, carbon monoxide gas)
- Exposure to blood or other bodily fluids

Managing a Motor Vehicle Collision Incident

A common scenario you may encounter is a motor vehicle collision with injured victims. Motor vehicle crashes are one of the leading causes of accidental death worldwide, especially among younger people. Although your first thought may be to help the victim(s), you must take steps to ensure the safety of yourself and other bystanders before rushing into the situation. If you witness a collision, do not perform any sudden dangerous maneuvers in your vehicle. Ensure that you park in a safe location without blocking access for emergency vehicles and switch on your hazard lights. If possible, wear high-visibility clothing and place an emergency warning triangle before the incident to warn other vehicles. All these steps will reduce the risk to yourself and other road users.

As well as moving vehicles, you should be aware of the other hazards in a motor vehicle collision. Vehicle fires are common, especially in a serious accident. There is a risk of explosion due to ignition of the fuel tanks. If the victim is in immediate danger from a fire, try to remove her from the scene if it is safe to do so. Otherwise, the victim should be kept as still as possible to reduce the risk of worsening potential neck and back injuries (see Neck and Back Injuries in Chapter 6). There may be broken glass or spilled fuel or oil around the damaged vehicles, so be careful before kneeling down to give first aid to a victim.

Finally, you should be aware of the risks of nondeployed airbags, especially in older vehicles. Airbags are lifesaving devices that can significantly reduce the chance of a fatal injury in a motor vehicle collision, especially if the collision is head on. If an airbag doesn't inflate during an accident, there is a risk it could deploy afterward. This could cause further injuries to the victim or to rescuers attempting to provide first aid to the occupants of the car. Always be aware of nondeployed airbags and try to avoid placing yourself in the path of the airbag.

Managing an Incident Near Open Water

Open water can be very dangerous, even if you're a strong and seasoned swimmer. The majority of accidental drownings occur in open-water scenarios. If a victim is in distress in the water, you should immediately summon help from emergency services or lifeguards. If possible, throw the victim an object such as an emergency life preserver to help him float. If the victim is near the shore, lie down and try to reach out to him with a stick or other long object. Never place yourself in harm's way; strong hidden currents can overcome even the most capable swimmer in a matter of seconds.

Managing an Incident Involving Fire and Smoke

Smoke and toxic fumes from a fire are as deadly as the hot flames. Do not enter a burning building; your safety is paramount. If you are in a building with an injured victim, attempt to evacuate her and yourself as quickly as possible. Do not stop to fight the fire or use fire extinguishers unless you are confident in using the extinguisher and the fire is small. Smoke will rise due to the heat; therefore, stay low and try to cover your nose and mouth to reduce the amount of toxic fumes you breathe in. If you become trapped, close all doors and place wet towels or clothing underneath the doors to minimize the amount of smoke that enters the room. Signal or call for help and await the arrival of rescue services. Anyone who has inhaled toxic smoke from a fire will require a medical checkup. The majority of deaths from fires are due to toxic smoke and burns to the airway and lungs. The dangerous effects of smoke inhalation can be delayed, and the victim may require a period of monitoring in the hospital.

Calling Emergency Services

As we discussed earlier in this chapter, your role is to provide initial care until the arrival of professional medical help. It is important when dealing with a first aid emergency to call for help early. The universal emergency number across North America (the United States and Canada) is 911. When you dial 911, you will be connected with an emergency operator who will ask a series of questions, including:

- The exact location of the incident
- The type of situation

- ■ The telephone number you are calling from
- ■ Specific details about the victim(s), the incident, and any potential hazards

When you dial 911, remain calm and answer the operator's questions as accurately as possible. The operator will use the details you give to prioritize the call and dispatch the appropriate emergency services. Some incidents may require more than one emergency service, especially if you have identified hazards. For example, a motor vehicle collision will likely require police, EMS, and fire and rescue to respond. If you have identified a hazard, then ensure you communicate this information to the 911 operator to allow her to plan the most appropriate emergency response.

If you are unsure of your location, then describe local landmarks or orient yourself using road signs. If you are calling from a landline, the 911 operator may already know your address, as information is passed automatically to the emergency call center.

The 911 operator may provide specific first aid advice over the telephone. For example, if the victim is unconscious and not breathing, the operator will guide you through performing cardiopulmonary resuscitation. You should follow the instructions the operator gives you. If you are calling from a mobile telephone that has a speaker function, use this to enable you to perform first aid while listening to the operator's instructions.

If traveling abroad, ensure you are familiar with the emergency contact number in the country you are visiting (see sidebar, Calling for Help Abroad).

Calling for Help Abroad

The following emergency numbers can be used to summon for help abroad:

- European Union: 112
- United Kingdom: 999
- Australia: 000
- New Zealand: 111

Protecting Yourself from Infection

You may encounter first aid situations in which there is a risk of exposure to blood or other bodily fluids. It is essential to have a basic understanding of infection control precautions to protect yourself and the victim from infection. Although they are not common, it is important to be aware of blood-borne viruses (viruses carried in the bloodstream). The three main blood-borne infections are HIV, hepatitis C, and hepatitis B. Blood-borne viruses can be transmitted if the infected blood crosses into the bloodstream of a healthy individual (for example, through a break in the skin or via accidental injection). Unless they are contaminated with blood, there is a very small risk of infection from other bodily fluids, including vomit, sweat, urine, and saliva.

Medical Terminology

HIV stands for *human immunodeficiency virus*. If left untreated, infection with HIV can cause *acquired immunodeficiency syndrome (AIDS)*.

However, these other bodily fluids can transmit other infections. For example, the influenza virus that causes the flu is transmitted via droplets produced when we sneeze or cough. Other viruses that cause diarrhea and vomiting (for example, norovirus) are transmitted via inadequate handwashing and sanitation.

You must always consider your safety when dealing with a situation in which there is a risk of coming into contact with bodily fluids. Assume all bodily fluids are infectious until proven otherwise. Always follow a set of standard precautions (see sidebar, Standard Infection Control Precautions) to protect yourself from the risk of infection.

Standard Infection Control Precautions

- Wear disposable gloves whenever there is a risk of contact with bodily fluid.
- If available, wear a disposable apron and eye protection.
- Wash your hands with soap and running water (see Appendix A: First Aid Techniques) or alcohol-based hand-gel if water is unavailable.
- Cover any cuts or grazes on your hands with a water-proof adhesive dressing.
- Dispose of contaminated medical waste and any needles appropriately.
- If available, use a disposable face mask when performing rescue breaths as part of cardiopulmonary resuscitation.

Protect Yourself with Infection Control Gear

All first aid kits should contain basic equipment to help you protect yourself from blood and other bodily fluids (see Appendix B: First Aid Kit Lists, for full suggestions). Even the most basic kit should contain disposable gloves to protect your hands and a face mask for performing CPR. Most disposable gloves are made of synthetic nitrile rubber rather than latex to reduce the risk of allergic reactions. If gloves are available, always wear them when there is a risk of contact with blood or other bodily fluids.

An apron and eye protection may be found in larger first aid kits. These items are useful to protect yourself from blood splashing in your eyes or on your clothing. For example, a severe wound may spurt blood, and there is a risk of infection if contaminated blood enters your eye.

Measuring Vital Signs

The four main vital signs are pulse (heart) rate, respiratory (breathing) rate, temperature, and blood pressure. These signs give us an indication as to how well the body is functioning and responding to an illness or injury. You should measure and document vital signs regularly before the arrival of EMS. The two signs you are most likely to measure are pulse rate and respiratory rate. EMS will carry equipment to perform more comprehensive vital sign monitoring, including measurement of body temperature and blood pressure. We will look briefly at pulse and respiratory rates.

Pulse Rate

The pulse is measured by feeling the beating of an artery. Each beat corresponds to the heart contracting and expanding, pushing blood through the body. While awaiting EMS you should record a pulse rate for all victims who are unwell. However, checking for a pulse is not recommended before deciding to commence cardiopulmonary resuscitation (CPR) in a patient who is not breathing, as this causes unnecessary delays. We'll explain this further in Chapter 3: Lifesaving Skills.

The pulse rate is recorded as the number of beats per minute (BPM). The pulse is often measured at the wrist by feeling the radial artery. It can also be found in the neck using the carotid artery, and in the elbow crease using the brachial artery.

The most accurate method to measure a pulse is to count the number of beats felt over one minute. However, to save time, it is acceptable to count for thirty seconds and double the result. Also, assess whether the pulse is regular or irregular. An irregular pulse may be a sign of an irregular heart rhythm. If you're unable to feel a radial pulse, attempt to feel a carotid pulse by placing two fingers on the victim's neck next to his windpipe. Do not attempt to feel both carotid arteries at the same time! The carotid arteries supply blood to the brain; if you compress both at the same time, you run the risk of cutting off this blood supply, and the victim will rapidly lose consciousness.

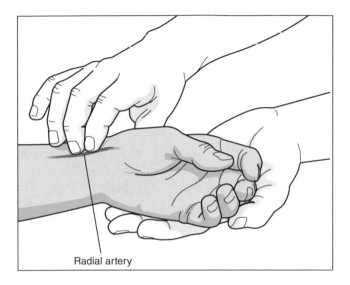

Radial artery

The radial pulse is felt at the inside of the wrist, just underneath the thumb.

Respiratory Rate

The respiratory rate is measured by counting how many breaths a person takes over one minute. However, once again, you can shorten this by counting for thirty seconds and doubling the result. To count the breaths, watch the chest rising and falling and count one for every completed rise and fall. You can also place a hand on the victim's shoulder or back to feel his breathing. Assessing an accurate respiratory rate can be challenging if the victim is wearing bulky clothing; garments might need to be removed if he's okay with you doing this. As well as counting the number of breaths, listen for any other sounds that may present when the victim breathes. There's no need to place your ear on his chest; you'll easily hear any abnormal sounds if they are present.

An asthma attack victim may be making a high-pitched wheezing sound when he breathes. Be mindful that telling a victim you are going to count his respiratory rate is likely to cause him to consciously alter his breathing pattern. By watching his breathing, you can also comment on his breathing pattern. For example, is he taking short, shallow breaths? Someone who is panicking or in pain may display this pattern of breathing.

Normal Pulse and Respiratory Rates

The normal, resting pulse and respiratory rates in adults are:

■ Pulse rate: sixty to one hundred beats per minute
■ Respiratory rate: twelve to twenty breaths per minute

These values may be affected by various individual factors, including age, physical fitness, medication, and clinical condition of the victim. For example, children have faster pulse and respiratory rates, whereas seasoned marathon runners often have a slower resting pulse rate.

Body Temperature

Measurement of body temperature requires the use of a thermometer. Mercury thermometers are no longer used, and many states have banned their sale due to health and environmental concerns. All thermometers in use now should be digital. Common sites to measure temperature include under the tongue, the forehead, the armpit, or in the ear (see sidebar, Measuring Body Temperature). A high temperature (fever) may be a sign of infection. If available, always record the temperature of an unwell adult or child. A normal body temperature is between 96.8°F (36°C) and 98.6°F (37°C), although this can vary slightly from person to person.

Measuring Body Temperature

Common sites to measure body temperature are:

- Under the tongue
- Inside the armpit
- Across the forehead
- In the ear

The location you use will depend on the model of thermometer you have. There are many varieties of digital thermometer available, and it is worth keeping one in a home first aid kit, especially if you have children. With young children, measuring temperature in the ear is normally the quickest and most effective method.

Blood Pressure

Blood pressure is measured with an automated blood pressure machine. There are both arm and wrist blood pressure monitors available, with many brands to choose from. Most blood pressure monitors will also record a pulse reading. The blood pressure is recorded as two numbers (for example, 130/80). The first number indicates the pressure in the blood vessels when the heart contracts. This is called the systolic blood pressure. The second, lower number is the pressure when the heart relaxes. This is called the diastolic blood pressure. Normal blood pressure in an adult is approximately 120/80. Persistent high blood pressure is known as hypertension and increases the risk of suffering a heart attack or stroke. A victim may take medications to lower her blood pressure (antihypertensives) to reduce this risk.

Watch the Trend

When recording vital signs, the overall trend is more important than one-off readings. For example, a rising heart rate in a victim with severe bleeding may indicate the victim is going into shock.

Record vital signs a minimum of every five to ten minutes in an unwell victim, and document your recordings to hand over to EMS.

Gathering Important Information from a Victim: AMPLE History

Gathering medical information from a victim is an integral part of first aid. Hand over this information to EMS when they arrive, since it may affect the victim's ongoing medical treatment. Also, it may help you determine what first aid treatment to provide. For example, a victim with difficulty breathing may tell you she carries an inhaler for her asthma or an EpiPen for a severe peanut allergy.

Finding out a victim's last oral intake is useful when dealing with diabetic emergencies (see Chapter 7: Medical Emergencies). A diabetic victim who has missed a meal is at risk of dangerously low blood sugar levels. In addition, if the victim requires emergency surgery, then knowing the time of his last meal or drink is helpful to assist hospital staff in planning the surgery.

Gathering information about the victim's medication is another important task. This information can affect the victim's ongoing care. For example, it is essential to establish whether a head injury victim is taking any blood-thinning medication (see Head Injuries in Chapter 6). Some people may carry alert cards or warnings related to specific medications that they take. This information should be handed over to EMS when they arrive.

You can use the acronym AMPLE to help you remember the important questions to ask a conscious and talking victim.

AMPLE Questions for a Conscious Victim

- **A**llergies: Do you have any known allergies to medication or food? Do you carry any medications to treat these, such as an EpiPen?
- **M**edications: What medication do you take from your doctor? Do you take any additional medication that you buy from a store?
- **P**ast medical history: Do you have any medical conditions? Have you had any recent surgery?
- **L**ast oral intake (food or fluid): When was the last time you had anything to eat or drink?
- **E**vents leading up to the incident: What happened prior to the incident or you becoming unwell?

Document the history provided and give the information to EMS when they arrive. If a victim is unconscious or unable to give you answers then you can ask any friends or relatives present to gather vital information.

Chapter Two
FIRST AID
EQUIPMENT GUIDE

FIRST AID KITS come stocked with a variety of dressings, bandages, and other supplies. You'll need to be familiar with the contents of a first aid kit and how to use the equipment properly. Different first aid kits contain different types and quantities of items, depending on the type of kit and where it is likely to be used. We've listed some suggested kit contents in Appendix B: First Aid Kit Lists. In this chapter we'll look at some of the common equipment you might find in all first aid kits. It is worth taking a moment to check the contents of your own emergency first aid kit. Do you know how to use each item?

Essential Equipment for First Aid Kits

All first aid kits should contain essential equipment in order to protect yourself in an emergency situation.

Infection Control

In Chapter 1, we explained how to protect yourself from infection in blood and bodily fluids. All first aid kits should contain basic protective equipment to reduce the risk of infection. At the most basic this should include disposable gloves to protect your hands. More comprehensive first aid kits should contain eye protection, disposable aprons, and equipment to safely clean up spills of blood or other bodily fluids.

The Complete First Aid Pocket Guide

Dealing with an emergency situation can be stressful. When under pressure, it can be hard to remember first aid treatments or signs and symptoms. All first aid kits should contain at least a basic quick guide to common emergency situations. When an emergency occurs, you can easily reference the quick guide and follow the steps to help the victim. Doing this removes the pressure of having to remember lots of information in an emergency situation. This book is a perfect companion to keep with any emergency kit!

Safety Equipment

Some larger first aid kits may contain safety equipment that is useful during an emergency. This could include basic items such as a flashlight and survival blanket for use during an outdoor emergency. Other items may include high-visibility clothing or emergency warning triangles for use during a motor vehicle collision. First aid emergency kits in the workplace may contain specialized safety equipment, such as a kit to deal with a chemical spill. This equipment should only be used by people trained and competent in managing hazardous situations.

Documentation

Finally, as we discussed in Chapter 1, you'll play an important role in gathering and recording information to pass over to EMS when they arrive. You need to record any information you gather from a victim, such as his or her allergy status or list of prescribed medication. Any vital signs that have been recorded should be documented and passed on to EMS. All first aid kits should come with a way of recording information. The most basic kit may only contain a pencil or a pen and a notepad. More comprehensive kits and workplace first aid kits may contain specific first aid report forms that you should complete for each victim and incident.

Wound Dressings

A first aid kit should contain equipment to deal with wounds of all sizes, ranging from minor cuts to life-threatening major bleeding. Let's look at some of the items you might find in a first aid kit.

Adhesive Dressings

Adhesive dressings or bandages are used to cover small cuts and wounds. They come in a range of sizes and shapes. Most of us have applied such a dressing at some point in our lives—the most common brand name for them is Band-Aid. An adhesive dressing provides protection for a wound and reduces the risk of infection. When applying one, it is important not to directly touch the pad as this will increase the chances of infection in the wound. Specialized dressings are used for blisters. These contain gel to cushion the blister.

Some people are allergic to the plastic or adhesive used in dressings. In this situation, use special low-allergy dressings. Alternatively, a small bandage or low-adherent dressing can be used instead of an adhesive dressing to cover the wound.

Low-Adherent Dressings

A low-adherent dressing is the pad of the bandage without any of the sticky adhesive. Like other bandages, low-adherent dressings come in a range of shapes and sizes. They are often used on wounds when the adhesive part of the dressing could cause further damage (for example, a large blister). Low-adherent dressings, as the name suggests, are designed not to stick to the wound itself. This is useful for victims with fragile skin and will reduce pain on removal of the dressing. All wound dressings are stored in sterile packaging, so it is important to minimize handling of the dressing before it is applied to the wound to reduce the risk of infection.

So how are low-adherent dressings secured in place? There are two options in this situation. The first is to use first aid tape to secure the dressing. This should be a plastic-free, paper-based tape so that it is suitable for use on people with allergies. However, tape can become loose and may not secure a dressing applied near a joint. In this situation, use a bandage (for example, an elastic bandage) to wrap around the low-adherent dressing and secure it in place. The bandage can be tied over the dressing, or tape can be applied to secure the bandage in place.

Pressure Dressing

A pressure dressing is used to cover a large wound and applies pressure to stop active bleeding. Pressure dressings consist of a sterile absorbent pad that is placed over the wound, and a stretchy "tail" of fabric that you wrap around the wound to apply pressure and secure the bandage. As well as stopping bleeding, these dressings also provide protection from infection. To provide the most effective pressure on the wound, tie the knot directly over the wound. Appendix A: First Aid Techniques, walks you through the steps of applying a pressure dressing to a bleeding wound.

Tourniquets

Tourniquets are now a standard item in trauma first aid kits—kits designed for use in a mass casualty incident. These specialized kits are now found in public buildings and transit stations across the United States. Evidence shows that victims can bleed to death from traumatic injuries (for example, a gunshot or stab wound) within minutes, well before the arrival of EMS or other first responders.

A tourniquet can be used to control major life-threatening bleeding from a limb and potentially save the victim's life. These are generally used as a last resort if the bleeding is not controllable with direct pressure over the wound. Purpose-made tourniquets are much more effective than improvised tourniquets. There are several brands of commercial tourniquets available. One of the most common you may encounter is the Combat Application Tourniquet (CAT). Take a look at Severe Bleeding in Chapter 6 for more detail on how to treat a victim who is bleeding.

How Does a Tourniquet Work?

A tourniquet works by cutting off blood flow to a limb by compressing the artery. If the tourniquet is applied effectively, the limb will not receive any blood at all, and the victim will not lose any more blood. Applying a tourniquet can be very painful for the victim. There is a risk of damage to the limb if the tourniquet is left on for a long time; this is why it is important to record when the tourniquet was applied. Some tourniquets have a label on which you can write the time they were applied.

Applying a Tourniquet

Tourniquets are applied approximately three inches above the wound. How a tourniquet is applied will depend on the type of tourniquet; many come with simple visual instructions that you can easily follow. Generally, most consist of a band that you wrap around the limb and then tighten with a rod (called a windlass) and secure in place.

Learn How to Stop the Bleed

The Stop the Bleed campaign run by the American College of Surgeons provides free training classes on how to help a victim who is bleeding profusely. These classes cover tourniquet basics and provide hands-on practice in their use.

You can find a class near you on the campaign's website, www
.bleedingcontrol.org.

Bandages

A first aid kit should contain a variety of bandages for creating
slings or strapping up a joint (for example, an ankle joint). Let's
look at some of the common bandages found in a first aid kit.
We've already discussed pressure dressings; these are bandages
used to control bleeding from a large wound.

Triangular Bandages

The most common item in a first aid kit used to make a sling
is a triangular bandage. This bandage is triangular in shape, as the
name suggests, and often manufactured from woven fabric. The triangular bandage can be used to make an arm sling for a victim with
a broken arm, wrist, or shoulder. Appendix A: First Aid Techniques,
walks you through the steps of making an arm sling from a triangular bandage. A first aid kit should contain a method of securing
the triangular bandage in place: either a safety pin or first aid tape.

Elastic Bandages

Elastic bandages are stretchable bandages used to support
a joint following a sprain or a strain (see Soft-Tissue Injuries in

Chapter 4). These bandages are wrapped around a joint and provide compression and support to the joint. The ankle is a commonly injured joint, and Appendix A: First Aid Techniques, will show you how to strap up an injured ankle using an elastic bandage. Elastic bandages can also be used to secure low-adherent dressings in place.

CPR Aids

Most first aid kits contain aids to assist you in performing cardiopulmonary resuscitation (CPR) on a victim who is unconscious and not breathing. CPR involves the delivery of chest compressions and optional rescue breaths to a victim (see Chapter 3: Lifesaving Skills). If you are trained and willing to give rescue breaths, use a barrier between yourself and the victim to reduce the risk of infection. There are two main types of barriers that you might find in a first aid kit: a resuscitation face shield or a pocket mask.

Resuscitation Face Shield

A face shield is a plastic film placed over the face of a victim who is unconscious and not breathing. The film has a valve that is positioned over the victim's mouth. This valve allows you to breathe air into the victim's lungs (rescue breaths) and prevents blood or vomit from coming into contact with your lips or mouth.

Resuscitation face shields are single use and should be disposed of after being used.

Pocket Mask

A pocket mask is a plastic mask placed over the victim's face when delivering rescue breaths as part of CPR. The mask contains a mouthpiece and a one-way valve to allow you to inflate the victim's lungs. In order for a pocket mask to be effective, there must be a good seal between the mask and the victim's face. Otherwise the air you blow into the mask will leak out the side, rather than going into the victim's lungs. Pocket masks can be tricky, as making a seal over the victim's face can be difficult. If you might be using a pocket mask, it is recommended to sign up for a practical first aid and CPR course, so you can have hands-on instruction and practice.

Chapter Three
LIFESAVING SKILLS

CARDIOPULMONARY RESUSCITATION (CPR) is one of the most well-recognized first aid techniques. However, did you know that the "kiss of life" is no longer required when performing CPR? First aid and CPR guidelines have changed dramatically over the past few years, and there is now a much greater emphasis on giving high-quality chest compressions. In this chapter, we'll describe the latest lifesaving first aid techniques to help a victim in cardiac arrest or during a choking emergency. The contents of this chapter could help you to save a life! We will start off by showing you how to assess an unresponsive adult victim, then how to perform CPR and use a defibrillator to help a victim of cardiac arrest. Finally, we'll discuss choking and how to perform the Heimlich maneuver on a choking victim. We'll be focusing on adult victims in this chapter; for children and babies take a look at Chapter 8: Pediatric Emergencies and Illnesses.

Assessing a Collapsed Victim

If you encounter a victim who has collapsed, you will need to act quickly to assess the situation and provide the appropriate first aid measures. A useful way to remember how to approach this situation is by using the DR ABC action plan. This action plan gives a structured way for you to assess the collapsed victim and remember what emergency action to take.

DR ABC Action Plan
DR ABC stands for:

- Danger
- Response
- Airway
- Breathing
- CPR

Let's take a closer look at the individual steps of the DR ABC action plan and find out how you could save a victim's life.

Danger
The first step (Danger) is to check for any potential hazards that could pose a risk to yourself, bystanders, or the victim. Quickly

assess the scene and ensure it is safe for you to approach. If you identify any hazards, take steps to reduce the risk of harm to yourself or bystanders (see Managing an Incident in Chapter 1). If available, wear disposable gloves in case of exposure to blood or other bodily fluids. Remember, you are the most important person in any emergency situation, and you are of no help if you become a second victim!

Response

Next, check for a response from the victim. Shout in both of her ears and firmly tap her shoulders. If you do not receive a response, then the victim is unconscious (see sidebar, What Is Unconsciousness?). This is a medical emergency, and at this point, you should call EMS if this has not been done.

What Is Unconsciousness?

If someone does not wake up when stimulated, then he is unconscious. An unconscious victim does not have an awareness of his surroundings or the events going on around him. This state is similar to being asleep, but the difference is that you can wake a person from sleep whereas an unconscious victim will not wake up.

Common Causes of Unconsciousness

- Cardiac arrest
- Severe head injury
- Fainting (temporary loss of consciousness)
- Low blood sugar levels
- Stroke
- Poisoning or intoxication
- Seizures
- Shock
- Hypothermia or heatstroke

Airway

The next step in the DR ABC action plan is to open the victim's airway. An unconscious victim is at risk of blocking his airway due to the tongue falling back and preventing air from flowing in and out of the lungs. Let's take a look at why this occurs and what you can do about it in first aid.

The airway refers to tubes and structures that air has to pass through to reach the lungs. The airway is at risk of becoming blocked if a victim is unconscious. When a victim loses consciousness, his tongue becomes very floppy, falls backward in his throat, and can block his airway. When this happens, no air can reach the lungs. This situation can quickly result in death.

To open the airway, place one hand on the forehead and tilt the head backward. Place your other hand underneath the bony part of the chin and lift the chin upward. This maneuver is known as a *head tilt chin lift* and will move the tongue away from the back of the airway, enabling the victim to breathe.

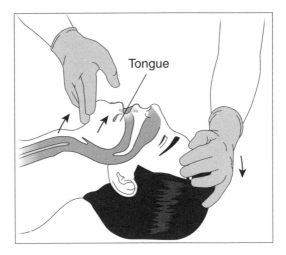

Tongue

The head tilt chin lift moves the tongue away from the airway at the back of the throat.

If you suspect the victim may have a neck or a back injury, then the jaw thrust maneuver should be used instead. In this technique, the head is not tilted backward, so there is less movement of the victim's neck. Take a look at Neck and Back Injuries in Chapter 6 for how to perform a jaw thrust and manage an unconscious victim with a possible neck or back injury.

Breathing

After opening the victim's airway, check for regular normal breathing for a maximum of ten seconds. To do this, place your cheek just above the victim's mouth and look at her chest. Feel for exhaled air on the side of your cheek, look for the chest rising and falling, and listen for the sounds of breathing. The occasional, infrequent gasp is not normal breathing and should be treated as no breathing. Infrequent gasping is known as agonal breathing and occurs in victims immediately following cardiac arrest (when the heart stops beating).

CPR

Now that you've assessed for danger and victim response, opened the airway, and checked the victim's breathing, there are two different situations for you to consider. The most important decision you need to make is whether to commence cardiopulmonary resuscitation (CPR). This is the last step in the DR ABC action plan.

The Victim Is Not Breathing Normally

If the unconscious victim is not breathing normally, then immediately commence CPR (see Cardiopulmonary Resuscitation (CPR) later in this chapter). It is vital that the 911 operator be kept informed of the victim's condition. Emergency services must be notified if the victim is not breathing so they can arrange an appropriate emergency medical response.

The Victim Is Breathing Normally

If the victim is breathing normally, perform a quick check to see if there is any major life-threatening bleeding. If you don't suspect a neck or a back injury, the victim should be rolled into the recovery position (see The Recovery Position later in this chapter) to further protect his airway.

Should I Check for a Pulse?

Studies have found that, in an unconscious patient who is not breathing, checking for a pulse is frequently inaccurate. In such a stressful situation you can often feel your own pulse through your fingers and mistake this for the victim's pulse. Additionally, you could be spending a long time trying to locate a pulse when actually it's not there or too weak to feel. Therefore, checking for the presence of a pulse during an initial assessment of a victim who is unconscious and not breathing normally is no longer recommended.

The Recovery Position

The recovery position, also known as the safe airway position, involves the victim being rolled onto his side in order to protect his airway and maintain effective breathing.

If you don't suspect a neck or a back injury then an unconscious but breathing victim should be placed in the recovery position to protect his airway. If you do suspect a neck or a back injury, then you should not move the victim unless you are unable to keep his airway open in the position in which he's found. Take a look at Neck and Back Injuries in Chapter 6 for more guidance on dealing with this situation.

Why is the airway so important? A victim who is unconscious is at risk of blocking his airway as we discussed in the previous section. The tongue can fall back and obstruct the airway, preventing air from flowing into the lungs. In addition, an unconscious victim is at risk of choking on his own vomit. At the entrance to the stomach is a muscle that prevents backflow of stomach contents up the gullet and into the throat. When you're unconscious, this muscle relaxes, and therefore stomach contents are free to flow up the gullet into the throat and then down into the airway and lungs. To reduce this risk with the help of gravity, an unconscious person should be rolled onto his side into the recovery position. In this position, any stomach contents will flow out of the victim's mouth and away from his airway.

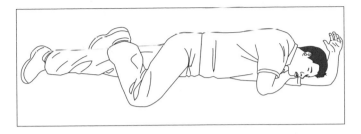

The victim is on his side to reduce the risk of choking on his vomit.

There are different methods for placing a victim in the recovery position, and no one method is superior. The victim should be on his side with no pressure on the chest wall to obstruct his breathing.

Rolling a Victim Into the Recovery Position

This version of the recovery position minimizes movement of the head and neck in case of a potential neck injury.

1. Kneel by the side of the victim.

2. Lift the victim's arm that is farthest away from you and place it above the victim's head with the palm facing upward toward the sky.

3. Place the victim's arm closest to you by her side.

4. Lift the victim's knee closest to you and place her foot flat on the floor.

5. Slide your arm that is closest to the victim's head underneath her shoulder blade and with that hand support her neck.

6. Roll the victim away from you by pushing on her shoulder; use your forearm with your hand supporting her neck, and use your free hand to push on her knee. Do not roll the victim by applying pressure to the head or neck.

7. As the victim rolls over, the head is cushioned by rolling onto her outstretched arm with your hand supporting her neck.

8. Ensure the airway is open and no pressure is on the chest wall.

9. Recheck her breathing to ensure she is still breathing normally.

Once the victim is safely in the recovery position, ensure EMS is called. Monitor vital signs and provide reassurance until emergency help arrives. If the victim stops breathing, update EMS and roll her onto her back to commence immediate cardiopulmonary resuscitation.

Cardiopulmonary Resuscitation (CPR)

An unconscious victim who is not breathing normally is likely to have suffered cardiac arrest. This occurs when the heart suddenly stops pumping blood through the body. Cardiac arrest is not the same as a heart attack (see Heart Attack in Chapter 7). However, a heart attack may cause cardiac arrest. Other causes of cardiac arrest include congenital (from birth) heart problems, significant blood loss, drowning, and poisoning. But what exactly happens to the heart during cardiac arrest?

Medical Terminology

The most common type of disorganized electrical activity that results in cardiac arrest is called *ventricular fibrillation (VF)*. *Ventricular* refers to the large chambers of the heart responsible for pumping blood, and *fibrillation* refers to the disorganized electrical activity. During ventricular fibrillation, the cells in the heart muscle do not contract in a coordinated way. This stops the heart from beating effectively as a coordinated unit, and blood stops flowing through the body.

The heart is a muscle responsible for pumping blood through the body. The heart is controlled by electrical activity that passes through the heart muscle and causes a coordinated heartbeat. The most common reason for cardiac arrest is the electrical activity in the heart becoming disorganized and chaotic.

During cardiac arrest, the heart is no longer pumping blood through the body. Our blood carries oxygen, which is vital to keep our cells and tissues alive. Brain cells depend on a continuous oxygen supply and will start to die after three to four minutes without oxygen. Brain cell death leads to permanent brain damage and reduces the chance of successful resuscitation from cardiac arrest.

Cardiopulmonary resuscitation (CPR) involves delivering chest compressions and, if you have been properly trained, rescue breaths to a victim of sudden cardiac arrest. The purpose of CPR is to push oxygenated blood through the body and keep the vital brain cells alive until the heart can start beating again. In effect, you take over the job of the victim's heart and lungs and become her life-support machine. That's why CPR is sometimes referred to as basic life support (BLS). CPR alone will not restart the victim's heart; it only buys time until the arrival of a device called a defibrillator (see Using an Automated External Defibrillator later in this chapter). The most important component of CPR is the delivery of effective chest compressions to a victim. It is now thought that rescue breaths are much less important, especially in the initial minutes following cardiac arrest, as the victim's blood will still be carrying some oxygen.

How to Perform CPR

Let's look at how to perform CPR on a victim of sudden cardiac arrest. We have already assessed danger, response, airway, and breathing, and established that the victim is not breathing normally. You must ensure that EMS has been called and then begin chest compressions.

For untrained bystanders, the American Heart Association now recommends performing chest compressions only and not stopping to attempt rescue breaths. High-quality chest compressions are the most important part of CPR, and it is vital that they are started quickly.

How to Give Effective Chest Compressions

To deliver high-quality chest compressions:

1. Kneel at the victim's side, parallel to his chest.
2. Place the heel of one hand in the middle of the victim's chest over the breastbone.
3. Place your other hand on top so your hands are parallel.
4. Push down to a depth of at least two inches (five centimeters).
5. Fully release and let the chest wall recoil.
6. Repeat and aim for 100 to 120 chest compressions per minute (maximum of two chest compressions per second). (The Bee Gees' song "Stayin' Alive" will help with timing.)

Keep your elbows locked and use your upper body weight to deliver effective chest compressions. Ensure that you let the chest wall recoil fully after each compression and do not lean on the victim's chest.

The delivery of effective chest compressions requires a significant amount of energy from the rescuer. Evidence shows that chest compression quality decreases after only one to two minutes of CPR. If more than one rescuer is available, trade performing CPR every one to two minutes.

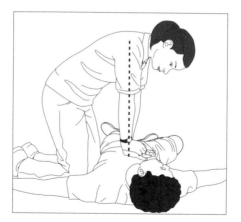

The proper technique for delivering chest compressions to a victim of sudden cardiac arrest.

Don't Worry About Rib Fractures

It is common for effective chest compressions to cause fractures of the victim's ribs and sometimes even his breastbone (sternum). Around a third of victims who receive CPR will sustain at least one rib fracture. If you feel rib fractures when performing CPR, recheck your hand position and the depth of chest compressions and continue performing CPR until EMS arrives. It can be off-putting if you hear or feel a rib fracture during CPR, but remember, you could save the victim's life. Any rib fractures you cause can be treated at a later date, but only if the victim is alive!

How to Give Effective Rescue Breaths

If you are a trained rescuer and willing to deliver rescue breaths, then perform two rescue breaths after each set of thirty compressions. Continue this cycle of thirty chest compressions to two rescue breaths.

1. Open the victim's airway by tilting the head backward.

2. Pinch the nose to prevent air leaking out.

3. Take a regular breath and make a seal over the victim's mouth, using a disposable resuscitation face shield if available.

4. Breathe into the victim's mouth for approximately one second; do not overinflate the victim's lungs as this

could cause air to go into the stomach and the victim to vomit.

5. Deliver two rescue breath attempts in total, then immediately resume chest compressions.

If two trained rescuers are present, one can perform chest compressions, and the other deliver rescue breaths, still at a ratio of thirty chest compressions to two rescue breaths. This two-person technique minimizes any interruptions in chest compressions.

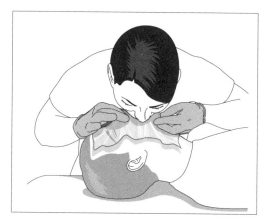

Pinch the victim's nose and tilt the head backward
to deliver effective rescue breaths.

The Complete First Aid Pocket Guide

Continue providing CPR (either chest compressions only, or chest compressions with rescue breaths) until the arrival of a defibrillator or emergency medical help. If a defibrillator is available, attach it to the victim and follow the instructions (see Using an Automated External Defibrillator later in this chapter). When EMS arrives, they may ask you to assist by continuing chest compressions while they perform advanced medical interventions.

The victim may vomit when you are performing CPR. If this happens, don't panic. It does not mean that you've done anything incorrectly. As we saw in the previous section, an unconscious victim can lose control of his stomach contents and may vomit. If the victim vomits when you are performing CPR, turn him onto his side to allow the vomit to drain away from the airway. Then turn him back and resume CPR as quickly as possible.

When to Stop CPR

CPR needs to be performed continuously for it to be effective. Stop CPR only if:

- The victim shows signs of life and is breathing normally.
- EMS arrives and asks you to stop.
- The environment becomes too unsafe for you to remain on scene, and you cannot safely move the victim.

- You become physically exhausted and unable to continue. Remember you are the most important person in any emergency situation. If you become exhausted and bystanders are present, show them how to perform chest compressions so they can take over.

CPR in Special Circumstances

There are some special circumstances to consider when performing CPR. These situations may require you to change how you give CPR to a victim in cardiac arrest. The same basic principles apply: chest compressions are the most critical component of CPR, and you should focus on delivering high-quality chest compressions to all victims of cardiac arrest. Let's take a look at some of the special situations you might encounter.

Children and Babies
We'll cover how to perform CPR on a child or baby in Chapter 8: Pediatric Emergencies and Illnesses.

Pregnancy
During the later stages of pregnancy, the unborn child rapidly grows in size, and the womb (uterus) expands. When a pregnant woman is lying on her back, the size of the womb can compress the major

blood vessels in the abdomen. This reduces the blood flow to and from the heart. During cardiac arrest, this compression of the blood vessels can make chest compressions less effective.

When delivering CPR, your priority is to deliver effective chest compressions. If there is a bystander or other rescuer present, she can manually displace the womb to the left-hand side. This technique relieves pressure on the blood vessels in the abdomen and will improve the effectiveness of your chest compressions. If no bystander is present, you can try placing a rolled-up jacket under the right side of the back to tilt the womb to the left and improve blood flow to the heart.

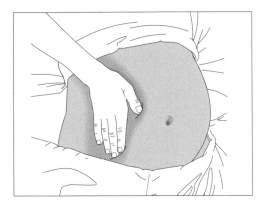

Moving the womb to the left-hand side will relieve
pressure on the abdominal blood vessels.

Confined Spaces

A cardiac arrest victim may collapse in a confined space, such as an airplane or in a restroom. If there is no space next to the victim to kneel and perform chest compressions, then deliver chest compressions using the over-the-head technique. Kneel at the victim's head with your knees almost touching his shoulders. Place your hands in the center of the victim's chest and deliver chest compressions.

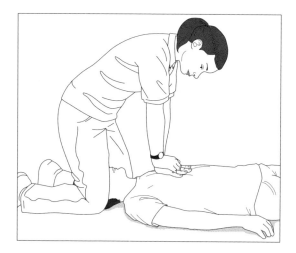

Over-the-head CPR can be used in a confined space.

The Complete First Aid Pocket Guide

Drowning

Victims of drowning are likely to vomit during resuscitation. Be prepared to quickly turn the victim to the side to allow the vomit to drain. If trained and willing, deliver rescue breaths after every cycle of thirty chest compressions. Remember your safety in a drowning situation—do not put yourself in danger and risk becoming an additional victim.

Victim on a Soft Bed

To be effective, chest compressions should be performed with the victim lying on a firm surface. If the victim is lying on a soft surface (for example, a mattress at home), the force you apply to the chest to perform compressions will just move the victim's body up and down and therefore the chest compressions will be ineffective. If possible, attempt to move the victim onto a hard surface before beginning CPR. Be mindful of your own safety, and do not perform any maneuvers that could cause you harm. If unable to move the victim, perform CPR in the position in which she was found and await the arrival of EMS.

Using an Automated External Defibrillator (AED)

A defibrillator is a medical device used to deliver a controlled electrical shock to a victim of cardiac arrest. As we have discussed, many cardiac arrests are due to chaotic electrical activity in the heart. The electrical shock from a defibrillator can clear this disorganized electrical activity and give the heart a chance to restore its normal rhythm, a bit like jump-starting a car. To be successful, a defibrillator needs to be used as soon as possible on a victim of cardiac arrest. Any delays will reduce the chance of restoring the heartbeat, even if adequate CPR is being performed.

An automated external defibrillator (AED) is a defibrillator designed to be used by bystanders with only basic medical training. An AED will analyze the victim's heart rhythm itself and only deliver an electrical shock if appropriate to do so. AEDs are highly effective devices if used promptly and are now an increasingly common feature in public places across the country, such as shopping malls and libraries. Many such places are now required by law to have an AED available and staff appropriately trained in its use.

If an AED is available nearby, it should be used as soon as possible once cardiac arrest occurs. There are many different models of AED on the market, and they will each have slightly different operating instructions. Most AEDs come with verbal and visual instructions. Once the device is switched on, it will guide the rescuer through how to operate the device and perform defibrillation. Follow these instructions carefully.

It is recommended that people using a defibrillator have basic practical training in CPR and using an AED. If your school, workplace, or gym has an AED, ask about whether practical training sessions are offered.

How to Use an AED

Here is how to use an automated external defibrillator:

1. Switch on the AED.

2. Expose the victim's bare chest.

3. Apply the electrical pads to the victim's chest as indicated by the instructions. If a victim has excessive chest hair you may need to remove this using a razor to ensure good contact of the pad with the skin. Warning! The pads are very sticky; if using gloves, take care that the pads don't become stuck together or to your gloves.

4. Follow the visual and audible prompts for the device. The AED will analyze the victim's heart rhythm and decide whether to deliver an electrical shock.

5. If the AED wishes to deliver a shock, ensure there is no one in contact with the victim before the shock is delivered. Give a loud verbal warning such as "*Stand clear!*" and press the shock button indicated on the machine.

6. Resume CPR if instructed to by the AED until the device gives you further instructions.

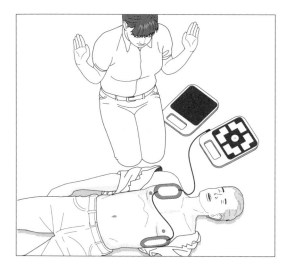

AEDs deliver a shock via electrical pads applied to the victim's chest.

The Complete First Aid Pocket Guide

The AED may deliver more than one electrical shock or instruct you to alternate between performing CPR and delivering shocks. Always follow the instructions from the AED until the arrival of emergency medical help. If possible, keep a record of how many shocks the AED has delivered and hand over this information to EMS.

AED Safety

An AED will deliver an electrical shock to the victim. There is a risk of harm if you or a bystander is in contact with the victim when the shock is given. Ensure no one is touching the victim before a shock is administered by the AED. The victim's chest should be dry to reduce the risk of burns. Most AEDs come with a small towel to dry the victim's chest if required.

Victims with Pacemakers

An AED can be used on a cardiac arrest victim with a pacemaker. Most pacemakers are located underneath the collarbone on the left-hand side. If you think a victim has a pacemaker, ensure the AED pads are not placed directly over the device.

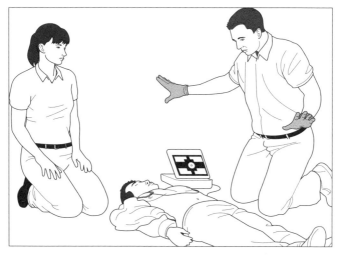

Give clear verbal and visual warnings to stand clear before the AED delivers a shock.

Helping a Choking Victim

Nearly everyone will suffer an episode of choking in his or her life-time. In the majority of cases it is mild, and a simple cough resolves the episode. However, choking can also be a life-threatening situation and without immediate first aid measures can result in cardiac arrest. In this section we'll talk you step by step through what to do if someone is choking and how you can help save his life.

Choking occurs when an object obstructs the airway and prevents air from flowing in and out of the lungs. If air (and therefore oxygen) cannot get into the lungs and therefore into the blood, it cannot be delivered to the tissues of the body, the most important being the brain and heart. If the heart does not receive an adequate supply of oxygen-rich blood, it will stop beating, leading to cardiac arrest. Choking is therefore a common cause of accidental death, especially in infants and the elderly. The most common object causing obstruction in this age group is food, but any small object can obstruct the airway. Children under the age of five are most at risk of choking as they have smaller airways and are at higher risk of swallowing objects they shouldn't. Staggeringly, around five thousand deaths occur each year in the United States due to chok-ing emergencies, and the majority of these deaths occur at home. But you can do something to help. Just keep on reading!

This section will cover how to help an adult choking victim. For children and babies see Chapter 8: Pediatric Emergencies and Illnesses.

The first aid treatment for choking involves the delivery of back blows and abdominal thrusts to attempt to dislodge the object and clear the airway. Abdominal thrusts are also known as the Heimlich maneuver. These two first aid techniques are not always effective in clearing an airway obstruction; therefore, do not delay in calling for emergency medical help for a choking victim. Chest thrusts are an alternative to performing abdominal thrusts.

Signs and Symptoms of Choking

- Clutching the throat or chest
- Difficulty in breathing
- Coughing
- Wheezing or grunting noises
- Red face initially, then turning pale or blue
- Reduced level of consciousness

If choking continues, the victim will become unconscious and stop breathing.

First Aid Treatment for Choking (Adult)

The first step in helping an adult choking victim is to establish whether there is complete or partial blockage of the airway. If the victim can speak and cough, then the blockage is only partial, as air is still able to move in and out of the lungs. If this is the case, then you should:

1. Encourage the victim to cough to dislodge the object.
2. Provide reassurance and monitor.
3. Loosen any tight clothing around the neck.
4. Call EMS if the symptoms do not quickly resolve.

If the victim is unable to speak or cough, then there is a complete obstruction of the airway. This is a life-threatening medical emergency. You should:

1. Immediately call EMS.
2. Deliver abdominal thrusts (Heimlich maneuver):
   a. Stand behind the victim and explain what you are going to do.
   b. Put your arms around his body, make a fist with one hand, and place this just above the victim's belly button.
   c. Grasp this fist with your other hand and firmly pull inward and upward. If unable to deliver abdominal thrusts, then deliver chest thrusts (see sidebar, Chest Thrusts) or back blows (see sidebar, Back Blows).
3. Continue giving abdominal thrusts, chest thrusts, or back blows until emergency medical help arrives.

4. If the victim loses consciousness, assess whether he is breathing normally. If he is not breathing normally, immediately update EMS and commence cardiopulmonary resuscitation (CPR) until the arrival of medical help (see Cardiopulmonary Resuscitation (CPR) earlier in this chapter).

Anyone who has suffered a serious choking episode should be assessed by a medical professional. Abdominal thrusts carry a risk of internal organ damage and bleeding, and therefore, these victims need an urgent medical assessment.

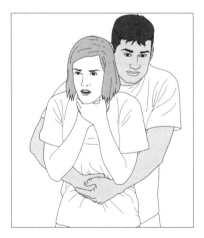

How to give abdominal thrusts.

Chest Thrusts

If you are unable to perform abdominal thrusts or the victim is heavily pregnant or obese, perform chest thrusts instead. To perform chest thrusts:

1. Stand behind the victim and explain what you are going to do.

2. Reach around and place one fist on the center of the breastbone (sternum).

3. Grasp this fist with your other hand and firmly pull inward.

4. After each chest thrust, check to see if the object has been dislodged.

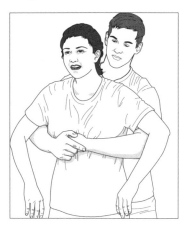

A heavily pregnant or obese victim may require chest thrusts instead of abdominal thrusts.

Back Blows

If you are unable to perform abdominal thrusts then back blows can be used to attempt to dislodge the object. To deliver back blows:

1. Lean the victim forward and explain what you are going to do.

2. Firmly hit him between the shoulder blades, using the heel of your hand.

3. After each back blow, check to see if the object has been dislodged.

Chapter Four
MINOR INJURIES AND CONDITIONS

THE MAJORITY OF FIRST AID SITUATIONS will involve treating victims with minor injuries and wounds. Thankfully, life-threatening emergencies such as a collapsed victim or severe choking are relatively rare, although it is important to know how to act in these situations! While minor injuries are not life-threatening, it is still important to have a good understanding of how to properly assess and provide appropriate initial first aid treatment for these injuries. Correct first aid treatment of a minor injury will reduce pain, speed up the healing process, and reduce the risk of long-term complications such as infection or scarring. Although these situations are not life-threatening, you need to be aware of the limitations of first aid and know when to seek professional medical help. In this chapter, we'll discuss a wide range of minor injuries and show you how to correctly assess and manage each injury. Let's start by looking at helping a victim with a minor wound, a very common situation that you will encounter.

Minor Wounds (Cuts and Grazes)

Cuts and grazes are common minor injuries in both adults and children. Our skin provides a protective barrier to prevent infection from entering our bodies. A minor wound causes a break in the skin, leading to the risk of infection entering the wound and potentially spreading into the bloodstream. First aid for minor wounds should focus on keeping the wound clean and preventing it from becoming contaminated with dirt or other sources of infection.

Many minor wounds can be cared for at home, using first aid measures without seeking medical attention. However, medical attention should be sought for deep or complicated wounds (see sidebar, When to Seek Medical Advice). Minor wounds will begin to heal within a day or so following the injury. If a wound doesn't start healing, you should seek medical advice as this could indicate a foreign body in the wound or the presence of infection.

When to Seek Medical Advice

You should seek urgent medical advice for a wound if you are concerned, or if any of the following situations apply:

- There is dirt or a foreign object in the wound (for example, a shard of glass)
- The wound is particularly deep
- The wound edges do not come together
- The wound has rough, jagged edges
- The wound is on the face; there is a risk of scarring
- There is any evidence of infection (see sidebar, Signs and Symptoms of an Infected Wound)
- The wound was caused by a bite from an animal or human
- The wound is a puncture wound
- The victim's tetanus immunizations are not up to date (see sidebar, Always Think About Tetanus)

Signs and Symptoms of an Infected Wound

- Pain
- A spreading red area around the wound
- Swelling
- Pus discharging from the wound
- High temperature (fever)
- Swollen glands near the wound

Do not delay seeking medical attention if you are concerned a wound is infected. If left untreated, the infection could spread to the bloodstream and cause blood poisoning (septicemia).

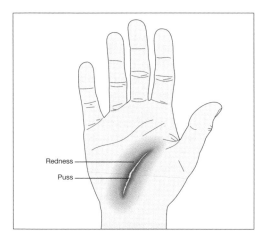

The signs of an infected wound.

First Aid Treatment for a Minor Wound

1. If the wound is bleeding, ask the victim to apply direct pressure to stem the bleeding.

2. Elevate the wound if it is on an arm or leg.

3. Wash your hands with soap and water (see Appendix A: First Aid Techniques) and put on disposable gloves.

4. Thoroughly wash the wound under running tap water. If running water is not available and you have a first aid kit, use antiseptic wipes to clean the wound.

5. If available, apply a topical antibiotic ointment or cream as long as the victim does not have any allergies to antibiotics.

6. Cover the wound with a sterile dressing to protect it from infection; small wounds may be covered with an adhesive dressing, while larger wounds may require a bandage.

7. Seek medical advice if concerned (see sidebar, When to Seek Medical Advice).

Tetanus is a severe infection caused by a germ that lives in soil and animal waste. The tetanus germ can enter the body through cuts and scrapes contaminated with dirt. Children are now routinely vaccinated against tetanus. Immunization requires multiple shots to be given, and some adults may require a booster if their last shot was more than ten years ago. Any victim with a dirty wound should be advised to seek medical attention for proper wound cleaning and an assessment of her or his tetanus risk.

Soft-Tissue Injuries (Sprains and Strains)

A soft-tissue injury occurs when there is damage to muscle, tendons, or ligaments. These structures are known as the soft tissues. Common soft-tissue injuries include sprains and strains (see sidebar, Medical Terminology, for the difference between a sprain and a strain).

Medical Terminology

A *sprain* occurs when there is damage to a ligament. Ligaments are tough bands of soft tissue that connect bones together. A *strain*, on the other hand, occurs when a muscle is overstretched, leading to damage to the muscle fibers or tendon. A tendon connects muscle to bone.

Soft-tissue injuries can occur due to abnormal twisting movements or the overstretching of muscles. These types of injuries are common among athletes; however, anyone can sustain a soft-tissue injury following a simple trip or fall at home. Soft-tissue injuries can be painful and cause a significant amount of swelling. Distinguishing between a soft-tissue injury and a broken bone is challenging, even for a medical professional. In first aid, you should not attempt to diagnose the type of injury the victim has sustained. All severe soft-tissue injuries should be evaluated by a medical professional who can provide a thorough assessment, including an X-ray of the injury.

Signs and Symptoms of a Soft-Tissue Injury

- Pain on movement of the area
- Tenderness
- Bruising and swelling (may not develop immediately)
- Muscle cramps or spasm
- Reduced joint mobility

First Aid Treatment for a Soft-Tissue Injury

You can remember the correct first aid treatment for a soft-tissue injury by using the acronym PRICE:

1. **P**rotect the area from further injury.
2. **R**est the injury.
3. **I**ce the injury to reduce swelling and pain.
4. **C**ompress the injury gently with a bandage or joint support.
5. **E**levate the limb to reduce swelling and pain.

Ice should not be applied directly to the skin as doing this can cause freeze burns. Many varieties of commercial ice packs are available. Only apply ice for a maximum of fifteen to twenty minutes at a time.

Severe soft-tissue injuries can cause significant damage to a joint and take several weeks to start healing. It is important to seek advice from a qualified medical professional regarding evaluation, rehabilitation, and physical therapy, especially if the victim is planning to return to an athletic activity. In rare cases, surgery may be required for severe or recurrent sprains.

Splinters

A splinter occurs when a small fragment of a large object becomes embedded in the skin. As anyone who works outside knows, wood splinters are common, although glass, metal, and plastic can also cause splinters. All splinters should be removed as soon as possible after they occur, as they can migrate farther into the body tissues and cause swelling or infection. Small splinters are often easily removed at home using tweezers; however, deep splinters or splinters that have been embedded for a period of time will require medical assistance to remove properly.

Signs and Symptoms of a Splinter

- Visible embedded object
- Puncture wound
- Pain
- Swelling around the area
- Signs and symptoms of infection (see Minor Wounds earlier in this chapter)

First Aid Treatment for a Splinter

Only attempt to remove superficial splinters. Seek urgent medical attention for deep or complicated splinters.

1. Clean the area with running water.

2. Put on disposable gloves.

3. Using clean tweezers (ideally a sterile, disposable set), attempt to remove the splinter back along the same angle at which it entered the skin.

4. After removing the splinter, clean the area again and cover with a sterile dressing.

Seek medical help if you are unable to remove the splinter, you have concerns that there is still an object embedded in the wound, or the area shows signs of infection.

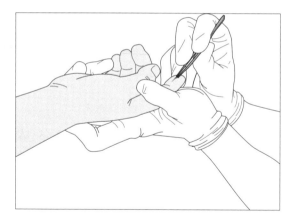

Remove a splinter back along the angle at which it entered the skin.

Wood Splinters and Tetanus

There is a risk of tetanus from wood splinters. Seek medical advice if the victim has sustained a wood splinter and her tetanus immunizations are not up to date or she is unsure about her tetanus immunization history.

Blisters

A blister occurs when a pocket of fluid forms in the superficial layer of the skin. This fluid causes a bulge underneath the skin. Excessive friction on the skin commonly causes blisters (this may occur as the result of wearing ill-fitting shoes, for example). The hands and feet are most prone to developing blisters, but they can occur on any part of the body. The fluid produced by a blister is designed to cushion and protect the underlying skin from further damage and aid healing. Bursting a blister will remove this protective layer and also increase the risk of infection developing (see sidebar, Don't Burst Blisters).

First Aid Treatment for a Blister

1. Clean and dry the affected area.
2. Cover the blister with a sterile dressing or specialized blister bandage. Don't apply the adhesive

directly over the blister, as this will cause damage when the dressing or bandage is removed.

3. Seek medical advice if the blister shows signs and symptoms of infection.

4. It is generally advised not to burst blisters (see sidebar, Don't Burst Blisters). If a blister bursts by itself, ensure the area is cleaned and covered with a sterile dressing to prevent infection.

It is always better to prevent a blister from occurring in the first place. Simple steps such as wearing the correct footwear can reduce the chances of developing a blister. If you feel an area of friction when walking (for example, on the heel of the foot), you can apply a bandage over the area to protect the skin and prevent a blister from developing.

Don't Burst Blisters

Blisters, like open wounds, cause a break in the protective layer of the skin and are at risk of becoming infected. For this reason, it is advised not to burst blisters as this will create a route of entry for harmful germs. If a blister shows signs of becoming infected, seek medical help.

Foreign Body in the Eye

Our eyes are delicate and vulnerable to contamination from foreign bodies such as grit, dust, metal, and other small objects. Wearing appropriate eye protection is essential when carrying out tasks that may cause eye injuries. A foreign body in the eye can cause permanent damage to the victim's vision and increase the risk of infection developing in the eye. Superficial foreign bodies that have not penetrated into the eyeball can often be washed out with running water or eyewash (see Appendix A: First Aid Techniques). If the surface of the eye is damaged or has been penetrated by the object, then specialist medical help will always be required to prevent loss of sight. A foreign body in the eye can scratch the surface of the eye (known as the cornea) and cause symptoms for several days after the object has been removed. Our eyes are precious and damage to vision can have serious long-term consequences for a victim. It is always best to seek advice and undergo a professional eye examination to ensure the foreign body has not damaged the eye.

Signs and Symptoms of a Foreign Body in the Eye

- A gritty sensation when blinking
- Pain, worse when moving the eye
- Eye watering
- Bloodshot eye
- Visual disturbance or loss of vision

First Aid Treatment for a Foreign Body in the Eye

1. Attempt to flush out the object using running clean water or sterile eyewash solution (see Appendix A: First Aid Techniques).

2. Do not rub the affected eye or attempt to remove the object with tweezers or a cotton swab.

3. If the object is large or sharp or you are unable to remove it quickly, seek medical advice.

Seek urgent medical attention if the object appears to have penetrated the eyeball or there are any problems with vision.

Watch Out for Arc Eye

Arc eye (also called welder's flash) is a painful eye condition caused by exposure to ultraviolet (UV) light from welding. The UV light causes a flash burn to the back of the eye, and the symptoms can mimic a foreign body in the eye with pain and a gritty sensation. Medical assistance is required in order to examine the eye carefully and antibiotic drops may be needed to prevent an infection from developing.

Knocked-Out Teeth

A blow to the face or mouth can result in an adult tooth becoming dislodged and falling out. A knocked-out adult tooth is a dental emergency and requires prompt treatment from a dental professional in order to save the tooth. Be aware that other injuries may exist in a victim with a knocked-out tooth. A direct blow to the face or the jaw can cause a fracture to the bones in the face. When dealing with a knocked-out tooth, your main aim is to try to save the tooth to enable its reimplantation by a dentist.

The best place for a knocked-out tooth is back in the socket; however, if this is not possible, then milk can be used to preserve the damaged tooth. In some cases, a knocked-out tooth can be swallowed or even go into the victim's airway. If this occurs, the victim will need urgent medical assistance in order to find and remove the tooth.

First Aid Treatment for a Knocked-Out Tooth

1. Hold the tooth by the upper half (crown). Do not touch the bottom half (root) of the tooth.

2. If the tooth is visibly dirty, briefly wash with running water; however, do not scrub the tooth or use soap.

3. If possible, place the knocked-out tooth back into the socket. Do not force the tooth in if you feel resistance or the victim experiences significant pain.

4. If unable to replace the tooth, place it in cold milk to preserve it until dental help can be sought.

5. If cold milk is not available, place the tooth in cold water, although this is less effective than milk in preserving the tooth.

6. Seek emergency dental help as soon as possible to give the victim the best chance of having the tooth reimplanted.

Nosebleeds

Nosebleeds are common in both adults and children. Our noses have a rich blood supply that helps warm the air we breathe in. Nosebleeds can occur spontaneously or following irritation or trauma to the nose. People who take blood-thinning medications are more at risk of developing nosebleeds and these nosebleeds can be difficult to stop. If a nosebleed does not stop after twenty minutes, seek medical attention; the blood vessel causing the nosebleed will need to be treated to stop further bleeding. In addition, although rare, recurrent nosebleeds can be a sign of a more serious underlying medical problem and should be investigated by a medical professional.

Rarely, a serious nosebleed can be life-threatening and can lead to shock from excessive blood loss (see Shock in Chapter 6). Always be aware of the potential for shock, and call EMS if the bleeding is uncontrollable or the victim goes into shock. Victims who take medication to thin their blood (see sidebar, Blood-Thinning Medication) are more at risk of having a serious nosebleed and requiring medical intervention to stop the bleeding.

First Aid Treatment for a Nosebleed

1. Lean the victim forward.
2. Ask the victim to pinch the soft part of the nose for a minimum of ten minutes without releasing.
3. If the bleeding is ongoing after the first ten minutes, ask the victim to reapply pressure for ten more minutes.

4. A cold compress or ice pack can be applied to the nose to reduce blood flow to the area.

5. If the nosebleed has not stopped after twenty minutes, seek urgent medical advice.

Once the nosebleed has stopped, the victim should not pick or blow his nose for at least twelve hours. If a victim has recurrent nosebleeds, then he should seek medical attention to investigate the underlying cause of the bleeding.

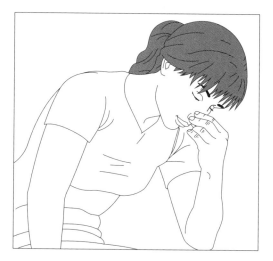

Pinch the soft part of the nose to stop a nosebleed.

The Complete First Aid Pocket Guide

Lean Forward Not Backward

Victims with a nosebleed should lean forward, not backward. By leaning forward, the victim will enable the blood to drain out the nose and not down into the throat. Leaning backward can cause the victim to swallow blood, and this can cause vomiting.

Blood-Thinning Medication

Some people take blood-thinning (anticoagulant) medication for heart conditions or following a blood clot. Examples of these medications include warfarin (Coumadin), rivaroxaban, apixaban, and dabigatran. These medications can make nosebleeds very difficult to stop, and the victim may require medical intervention to find and stop the bleeding blood vessel. Also, you should be aware that in patients taking warfarin, a nosebleed may be a sign of dangerously thin blood. These victims may need a blood test to check the warfarin levels and dose adjustment as necessary by a medical professional.

Fainting

Many of us have witnessed, or experienced, a fainting episode. So, what exactly causes someone to faint? Fainting occurs when the blood supply to the brain is temporarily interrupted. As a result, the brain does not receive enough oxygen or nutrients. This results in a temporary loss of consciousness, and the victim often falls to the floor. A victim of fainting usually recovers quickly once lying down, since being horizontal on the floor improves the blood supply to the brain, as the heart does not have to pump blood against gravity. There are many different causes of fainting (see sidebar, Causes of Fainting), and normally a victim will recover without any problems. Sometimes, recurrent fainting (especially during exercise) can be a sign of a more serious underlying heart condition and will require a checkup from a medical professional. In addition, victims of fainting can sustain serious injuries when they fall to the floor, especially if they are elderly. Always seek medical attention if you are concerned a victim is injured following a fainting episode.

Medical Terminology

The medical term for fainting is *syncope*.

Causes of Fainting

- Environmental trigger: unpleasant sight or smell or excessive heat
- Medication use
- Dehydration
- Abnormal heartbeat
- Underlying heart problem

Signs and Symptoms of Fainting

- Temporary loss of consciousness followed by a quick recovery
- Feeling weak, light-headed, or sick
- Pale, gray skin
- Sweating
- Presence of an external trigger that caused the faint (for example, the sight of blood from a nosebleed)

First Aid Treatment for Fainting

1. If a victim feels he is going to faint, advise him to lie or sit down as quickly as possible.

2. If he loses consciousness, raise his legs to improve blood flow to the brain.

3. The victim should quickly recover. If he does not, ensure the airway is open and he is breathing normally.

4. Check for any injuries if the victim has fallen.

5. Monitor vital signs and provide reassurance until the episode resolves. If you are concerned that the victim is not recovering, or the victim has sustained an injury, call EMS.

6. Advise the victim to seek medical attention to investigate the underlying cause.

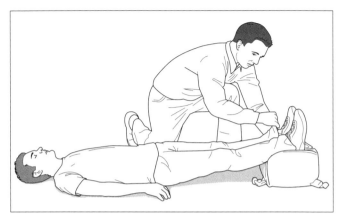

Raise the victim's legs to improve the blood flow to the brain
and help the victim recover after fainting.

Black Eye

A black eye occurs when there is bruising around the eye. Often, this occurs after a direct blow to the face; small blood vessels underneath the skin are damaged and blood collects there, causing swelling and bruising. Black eyes can look serious, but they often start to heal within a few days. You should be aware that a victim with a black eye may also have a head injury or fracture to the face and may require urgent medical attention for this (see Head Injuries in Chapter 6 for guidance on how to recognize and treat a serious head injury). It is important to check for any injury to the eye itself. If the eye is damaged, specialist medical attention will be required to prevent any permanent damage to the victim's vision.

First Aid Treatment for a Black Eye

1. Assess the victim for any evidence of a serious head injury (see Head Injuries in Chapter 6) or damage to the eye.

2. Clean and cover any open cuts or grazes.

3. Apply an ice pack or cold compress to the affected area to reduce the swelling; do not apply ice directly to the skin.

4. Seek medical advice if any concerning features are present (see sidebar, When to Seek Medical Advice).

When to Seek Medical Advice

Seek medical advice if you are concerned about a black eye, or if any of the following are present:

- Evidence of a serious head injury, such as loss of consciousness, seizures, or vomiting
- Significant swelling around the eye or intense pain
- Bleeding into the eye
- Loss of vision
- Inability to move the eyeball
- Evidence of infection, such as increasing pain, swelling, or redness around the black eye
- Use of blood-thinning medication (anticoagulants) by the victim

Don't Use Raw Meat

Using raw meat (such as steak) to speed up healing of a black eye is a first aid myth. There is no evidence that meat will aid healing, and it could worsen the situation by introducing infection into the eye. So, save yourself some meat and use a cold compress or ice pack instead!

Broken Nose

Injuries to the nose are common, especially when playing sports that involve close contact. It can sometimes be difficult to tell whether the nose is broken, or just badly bruised and swollen. If a broken nose is in the wrong position, it may need realignment by a medical professional. Rarely, a broken nose can lead to more serious damage to the nose or the underlying bones of the face. In some cases, surgery may be required to fix the break. If you are concerned about a suspected broken nose, always seek early medical attention. You should be aware that a victim with a broken nose may also have a head injury and he may require urgent medical attention for this (see Head Injuries in Chapter 6 for guidance on how to recognize and treat a serious head injury).

Signs and Symptoms of a Broken Nose

- Swelling around the nose
- An obvious deformity
- Pain and tenderness
- A cracking or grating sound when touching the nose
- Bleeding

First Aid Treatment for a Broken Nose

1. Assess the victim for any evidence of a serious head injury (see Head Injuries in Chapter 6).

2. Clean and cover any open cuts or grazes on the nose.

3. Apply an ice pack or cold compress to the affected area to reduce the swelling; do not apply ice directly to the skin.

4. Treat any nosebleeds by asking the victim to lean forward and pinch the soft part of the nose for a minimum of ten minutes (see Nosebleeds earlier in this chapter).

5. Seek medical attention; do not attempt to reposition the nose yourself, as you risk causing further damage.

Minor Burns

More than a million Americans each year require medical attention due to burn injuries. The majority of these injuries are minor burns and do not cause any serious complications. In this section we'll look at how to effectively treat a minor burn injury. If a victim has suffered major burns, she will need urgent medical treatment (see Major Burns in Chapter 6). A minor burn normally only affects the superficial layer of the skin. In some cases a small blister may form over the burn site.

Minor burn injuries can be very painful! Prompt first aid treatment can reduce the pain and swelling from a burn injury and speed the recovery process for the victim. You should be aware that all burn injuries are at high risk of becoming infected. This occurs because a burn causes a break in the skin, which is our protective barrier against germs. Always seek medical advice if you are concerned about an infected burn, as antibiotics may be required to treat the infection.

First Aid Treatment for a Minor Burn

1. Immediately cool the burned area for a minimum of twenty minutes with cool running water.

2. If possible, remove any rings, watches, or straps near the burned area before the burned area begins to swell.

3. Cover the burn loosely with a non-fluffy sterile dressing. Clean plastic wrap can be used if no sterile dressings are available.

When to Seek Help

Even minor burns may require specialist medical attention. The following situations always require medical assistance:

- The burn involves the face, feet, hands, or genital area
- There is any evidence of infection in the burn: increasing pain, redness, or discharge of pus
- The burn is located near a joint, such as the knee
- The victim is elderly or a very young child
- Large blisters have formed
- Rings or watches are stuck due to excess swelling around the burn

Common Minor Burn Injury Myths

There are many myths regarding the correct first aid treatment of burns. Many food products have been suggested as potential treatments for burns; however, it's best to keep the butter and mayonnaise in the fridge and use only water to cool a burn.

- Do not apply toothpaste, butter, or any other foodstuff to a burn. This will not cool the burn adequately. The best method to cool a minor burn is by using running water.
- Do not burst blisters; doing this will increase the risk of infection in the burn.
- Do not place ice on a minor burn to speed up the cooling process; the ice could make the injury worse by causing freeze burns to the skin.

Chapter Five
COMMON ILLNESSES

MOST COMMON MINOR ILLNESSES, such as earaches or headaches, can be managed at home with simple self-care measures. In this chapter, we'll discuss some of the most common illnesses and the correct first aid treatment in each situation. Generally, most first aid treatments for minor illnesses are supportive (for example, reducing pain and swelling) while the body fights off the infection or heals.

Most of the time medical attention is not required. However, in some situations a minor illness may be a sign of a more serious underlying medical problem. Always seek help if a minor illness does not appear to be resolving. **Remember that this first aid pocket guide does not replace professional medical advice!**

Earache

Earaches are a common problem, especially in children. The most common cause of earache is an infection, either in the outer part of the ear (the ear canal) or behind the eardrum (the middle ear). A foreign object lodged inside the ear can also cause an earache. The nerves that supply the ear also supply areas of the throat and teeth. Therefore, problems such as a toothache or a sore throat can sometimes cause pain in the ear.

Most causes of earaches can be treated at home with simple first aid measures. A severe ear infection may require antibiotics. If an earache does not resolve within a couple of days, medical advice should be sought as, very rarely, a persistent earache can be the sign of a more serious underlying medical problem or a problem in the mouth or throat.

First Aid Treatment for an Earache

1. Advise the victim to take regular over-the-counter painkillers such as acetaminophen.

2. Place a warm compress, such as a warm, wet washcloth, against the ear.

3. Seek medical advice if you are concerned, there is hearing loss, or the earache does not resolve.

4. If the eardrum has been perforated (see sidebar, Perforated Eardrum), keep the inside of the ear dry and avoid submersion in water.

Perforated Eardrum

Infection behind the eardrum can occasionally cause a tear in the eardrum. This is known as a perforated eardrum. Signs of a perforated eardrum include hearing loss and discharge from the ear. Normally, an eardrum perforation will heal by itself with time (around six to eight weeks). In rare cases, surgery may be required to repair the eardrum. Always seek advice from a medical professional, especially if there is significant hearing loss or discharge coming from the ear.

Diarrhea

Diarrhea occurs when bowel movements become loose, watery, and more frequent. Typically, when diarrhea occurs, you will have to have a bowel movement more than three times a day. There are many different causes of diarrhea; the most common cause of sudden-onset diarrhea in a victim is inflammation of the gut due to an infection.

The main risk from diarrhea is dehydration from passing large quantities of loose, watery stool. Young children and the elderly are most at risk of developing dehydration from diarrhea. In some cases, hospital admission is required for regular blood tests and fluid replacement through intravenous (IV) fluids.

Persistent diarrhea can sometimes be a sign of an underlying inflammatory disease affecting the bowel (for example, Crohn's disease or ulcerative colitis). Always seek medical advice if diarrhea does not resolve with simple first aid measures or if there is any blood visible in the stool.

First Aid Treatment for Diarrhea

1. Encourage the victim to drink fluids to prevent dehydration; commercially available oral rehydration solutions (ORS), which include essential salts and sugar, can be used.

2. Ensure you and the victim perform adequate hand-washing to reduce the risk of infection spreading.

3. Consider trying antidiarrheal medication (for example, loperamide) to improve symptoms.

4. Seek medical help if you are concerned that the symptoms are not resolving, there is blood in the stool, or the victim is displaying signs of dehydration (see sidebar, Spotting Dehydration).

Spotting Dehydration

The main risk from diarrhea is dehydration. The following warning signs may suggest a victim is becoming dehydrated:

- Excessive thirst
- Dry tongue and lips
- Tenting of the skin
- Increased pulse rate
- Lethargy
- Confusion

Always seek urgent medical attention if you are concerned that a victim is becoming dehydrated.

Nausea and Vomiting

Nausea and vomiting are unpleasant symptoms that we've all experienced at some point. The most common cause of sudden-onset nausea and vomiting is an infection in the stomach or gut (gastroenteritis). Other causes include poisoning, side effects of medication, severe head injuries, and severe pain. Most cases of nausea and vomiting should resolve within a day or so with simple first aid measures. Persistent nausea and vomiting should be investigated by a medical professional. Young children and the elderly are most at risk of developing dehydration from vomiting. In some cases, hospital admission is required for fluid replacement through an IV and anti-nausea medication to stop vomiting.

Vomiting up blood is a medical emergency and requires urgent investigation and treatment. Bleeding into the stomach or gut can be life-threatening if left untreated. The blood may appear bright red and fresh, or alternatively, it may be partly digested by the stomach. Partly digested blood is much darker and is often described as looking like coffee grounds. A victim who is vomiting lots of blood may go into shock. Be aware of this risk (see Shock in Chapter 6); closely monitor any victim who is vomiting up blood and check her vital signs at regular intervals until EMS arrives.

Medical Terminology

Nausea is the sensation of feeling sick. *Vomiting* is the active process of being sick.

First Aid Treatment for Nausea and Vomiting

The first aid treatment for nausea and vomiting is supportive. There's not much you can do in first aid to fix the underlying cause. Instead, your aim is to prevent the victim from becoming dehydrated and to seek early medical help if concerned.

1. Encourage oral fluid intake to prevent the victim from becoming dehydrated; commercially available oral rehydration solutions (ORS), which include essential salts and sugar, can be used.

2. Encourage the victim to sip fluids in small mouthfuls and often, rather than taking a large drink at one time. This reduces the chance that the victim will immediately vomit the fluid back up.

3. Ensure you and the victim perform adequate hand-washing to reduce the risk of infection spreading.

4. Call EMS if the victim is vomiting blood or has severe abdominal pain, or if you suspect the victim is severely dehydrated.

Morning Sickness

Morning sickness is very common during the early stages of pregnancy and is thought to be due to the high levels of pregnancy hormones traveling through the body. Morning sickness can be persistent and can lead to other medical problems such as dehydration or loss of essential salts and minerals from the body. Always seek medical assistance in the case of excessive morning sickness, as rehydration through an IV or strong anti-nausea medication may be required to deal with the unpleasant symptoms of morning sickness.

Common Cold

The common cold is an infection of the upper airways (nose, throat, and sinuses) caused by a viral infection. Viruses are tiny organisms that reproduce inside our cells and cause infections. The virus that causes a cold normally affects the lining of the nose, causing a runny nose and sneezing. This is also the way the cold virus spreads from person to person. Every time we sneeze, thousands of small droplets are produced and expelled at high speed across a wide area. These droplets carry the cold virus and can contaminate surfaces and infect people in the surrounding area. Catching sneezes in tissues and effective handwashing are important steps to take to reduce the spread of viruses that cause colds.

Unfortunately, there is no role for antibiotics in treating the common cold. Antibiotics are only effective against infections caused by bacteria, not viruses. Using antibiotics for the common cold is likely to cause side effects and can lead to the development of antibiotic-resistant organisms. Our bodies should fight off the cold virus within seven to ten days, although in some cases it can take several weeks for the infection to be completely resolved.

Medical Terminology

The virus responsible for causing most cases of the common cold is known as a *rhinovirus*.

Signs and Symptoms of the Common Cold

- Sore throat
- Runny and congested nose
- Sneezing
- Coughing
- High temperature (fever)

First Aid Treatment for the Common Cold

1. Advise the victim to take regular over-the-counter painkillers and antifever medication such as acetaminophen.

2. Encourage the victim to sip fluids to prevent dehydration.

3. Ensure you and the victim perform adequate hand-washing to reduce the risk of the infection spreading.

4. Seek medical help if you are concerned that the symptoms are not resolving, or if the victim may be suffering from influenza (the flu).

What About Cough Syrups?

Many people use commercial cough syrups to deal with the troublesome symptoms of a cold. However, scientific studies show that cough syrups may not provide much relief and, in some cases, may have harmful side effects (for example, drowsiness), especially if used in large quantities. Parents should be aware that cough syrups are not recommended for use in children due to the risk of side effects. The Food and Drug Administration (FDA) advises that children under the age of two should not be given any commercially available cough syrups.

Influenza (The Flu)

The influenza virus is responsible for causing a respiratory infection known as the flu. The flu is a highly contagious infection more common in winter months. The flu is more serious than a common cold, and vulnerable people (such as young children, the elderly, and people with long-term medical conditions) can suffer from serious complications. In some cases, the flu can be life-threatening and require hospital treatment, so always seek urgent medical assistance if you are worried about a victim with suspected influenza. Vaccination programs are designed to reduce the impact of the seasonal flu infection and provide protection for people; however, these vaccines do not provide guaranteed protection from catching the influenza virus.

The first aid treatment for influenza involves supportive care to ensure the victim remains well hydrated and treating any pain or fever. Flu symptoms can last around five to seven days, sometimes longer. There are now antiflu medications available, which can be prescribed by doctors. These medications may shorten the duration of flu symptoms in some individuals, but unfortunately, they do not cure the illness. These medications are normally recommended for patients at high risk of developing complications from flu (for example, elderly people or those with long-term breathing problems).

Signs and Symptoms of Influenza

- High temperature (fever)
- Headache
- Lethargy and fatigue
- Muscle aching
- Cough
- Sore throat
- Nausea and vomiting
- Diarrhea

First Aid Treatment for Influenza

1. Advise the victim to take regular over-the-counter painkillers and antifever medication such as acetaminophen.

2. Encourage the victim to sip fluids to prevent dehydration.

3. Ensure you and the victim perform adequate hand-washing to reduce the risk of the infection spreading.

4. Seek medical help if you are concerned that the symptoms are not resolving, the victim appears very unwell, or she or he develops other medical problems.

Headache

All of us have had a headache at some point in our lives. Most headaches, while an inconvenience, are not serious and resolve with no medical treatment apart from simple painkillers. However, there are some warning signs that you should be aware of, and we'll talk about them in this chapter as sometimes a headache can be a symptom of a more serious underlying medical problem. Many of the common illnesses described in this chapter (for example, the common cold) will cause headaches that will resolve as the illness improves.

Some people suffer from recurring headaches known as migraines. These are severe, unpleasant headaches often associated with other symptoms such as nausea, vomiting, and being sensitive to light or loud noises. Migraines can be very painful, and patients may be prescribed strong antimigraine medication to take when a migraine starts.

First Aid Treatment for a Headache

1. Advise the victim to take regular over-the-counter painkillers such as acetaminophen.
2. Seek medical advice if the headache does not resolve or any concerning features are present (see sidebar, When to Seek Help).

3. Call EMS if the victim has a reduced level of consciousness or any signs of meningitis (see Meningitis in Chapter 7).

When to Seek Help

Minor headaches are usually treated at home with simple painkillers. However, there are certain situations when you should seek medical help:

- Sudden-onset (in a split second) extreme headache
- Reduced level of consciousness
- Possible meningitis (see Meningitis in Chapter 7)
- Seizures
- Persistent headache not relieved by painkillers or associated with persistent vomiting
- Severe dizziness or visual loss
- Loss of memory (amnesia)

Motion Sickness

Motion sickness is an unpleasant feeling of nausea, sometimes with vomiting, caused by traveling in a car, boat, plane, or other moving vehicle. Some people seem to be more susceptible to motion sickness than others, although the reason for this is still unknown. So why does motion sickness occur?

Our brains sense movement in two main ways: our eyes and our ears. The eyes transmit information about the world around us to the brain. Our ears, as well as being responsible for hearing, also play an important role in letting the brain know about our position and movements. When these two senses become confused, motion sickness occurs. For example, when we are traveling in a car, our eyes can see that we are moving quickly; however, the inner ear does not pick up on this movement, and the brain receives mixed messages. This results in the unpleasant symptoms of motion sickness.

There are very effective medications now available for the prevention and treatment of motion sickness. Some of these medications may have side effects such as drowsiness so it is important to speak to a medical professional to choose a medication that is right for you.

Signs and Symptoms of Motion Sickness

- Nausea (feeling sick)
- Vomiting (being sick)
- Dizziness
- Headache
- Sweating

First Aid Treatment for Motion Sickness

1. Choose a forward-facing seat to prevent motion sickness. If traveling in a car or on a bus, try to request a seat in the front of the vehicle.

2. Avoid reading or using electronic devices.

3. Try to focus on a stationary object in the distance.

4. Avoid drinking alcohol or excessive caffeine.

5. Use anti–motion sickness medications. Remember, these can be associated with strong side effects such as drowsiness and fatigue.

Panic Attacks and Hyperventilation

A panic attack occurs when a victim experiences sudden intense anxiety, usually accompanied by physical symptoms such as hyperventilation (breathing too fast), sweating, palpitations (fluttery or rapid heartbeat), and muscle cramps. Panic attacks can be very frightening and may strike without warning. The physical symptoms associated with a panic attack can be severe; these symptoms often intensify the victim's anxiety state, and the panic attack worsens.

Hyperventilation, or overbreathing, is a common feature of panic attacks. In severe cases, this can lead to numbness or clawing of the hands and tingling of the lips. This occurs because overbreathing affects the level of carbon dioxide in the blood, which causes the symptoms of tingling, numbness, and hand clawing. These symptoms can make the victim more anxious and therefore worsen the hyperventilation and panic attack.

Always remember that hyperventilation may be due to another medical problem (for example, an acute asthma attack or a heart attack). If you are worried the victim is having a medical emergency, then call EMS.

People who have regular panic attacks may take antianxiety medication or carry medication to use when a panic attack strikes. Let's take a look at what you can do to help a victim of a panic attack.

First Aid Treatment for Panic Attacks and Hyperventilation

1. Remain calm and reassuring.

2. Ask the victim if there is anything you can do to help (for example, by removing a trigger of the panic attack).

3. Focus the victim's breathing—talk the person through taking deep, slow breaths to slow down hyperventilation.

4. Provide lots of reassurance and maintain the victim's dignity (for example, ensure any bystanders move on).

5. Call EMS if the victim loses consciousness, she appears to be having severe difficulty breathing, or you suspect she is having an asthma attack.

Avoid Using Paper Bags

Using a paper bag to control a panic attack victim's breathing is no longer recommended. Breathing into a paper bag will rapidly increase the amount of waste carbon dioxide in a victim's blood. If the victim is hyperventilating due to another medical problem such as a heart attack or asthma, this could be dangerous for her.

Chapter Six
TRAUMATIC INJURIES

AS WELL AS MINOR INJURIES, you may encounter a victim with more serious injuries such as severe bleeding or a head injury. Some of these injuries can be life-threatening and you need to know the correct steps to take if you find yourself looking after an injured victim. The actions you take in the first few minutes following a serious traumatic injury (for example, by applying pressure to a badly bleeding wound) could be lifesaving!

When dealing with traumatic injuries, remember to consider your own safety. Victims may have been injured in a motor vehicle collision or a fight. These can be chaotic and dangerous situations to enter. Always carry out an assessment of the scene and identify potential hazards before rushing in to help (see Managing an Incident in Chapter 1).

Let's start by looking at how you can help a victim who is bleeding profusely from a major wound.

Severe Bleeding

Our blood is responsible for carrying oxygen through our bodies and delivering it to our vital cells and tissues. Blood also removes waste products from cells and prevents the buildup of toxins. The average adult has around five liters of blood, although this depends on weight and size. Blood is transported through the body in three main blood vessels. Let's take a look at these in more detail and see what happens when they are damaged.

Arteries carry blood under high pressure away from the heart, veins carry blood under low pressure back to the heart, and capillaries are tiny vessels that deliver blood to the cells of the body. Injury to an artery will cause a wound to bleed quickly, since the blood in the artery is under high pressure. These wounds are serious and require urgent first aid steps to stem the bleeding. In some cases, the blood will spurt out of a wound due to the pressure in the artery. The blood in a vein is under less pressure, so blood will not spurt out. However, large veins carry lots of blood, and injuries to these will cause significant bleeding. Injury to the small capillaries causes blood to ooze from a wound; you often see this with small cuts and grazes.

Severe bleeding is an emergency situation, and losing too much blood is life-threatening for the victim. The main concern with severe blood loss is the victim going into shock (see Shock later in this chapter). Swift first aid treatment is vital to stopping or slowing the bleeding before the arrival of emergency medical help. When dealing with a severe bleeding situation, ensure you are aware of your own safety and take adequate precautions to protect yourself from blood-borne viruses (see Protecting Yourself from Infection in Chapter 1).

Medical Terminology

The medical term for bleeding is *hemorrhage*.

First Aid Treatment for a Major Bleed

1. Immediately call EMS.
2. Wear disposable gloves and apply firm, continuous, direct pressure over the bleeding point.
3. If the wound is on a limb, elevate the limb above the level of the heart to reduce blood loss.
4. If available, apply a sterile pressure bandage directly over the wound (see Appendix A: First Aid Techniques).
5. If direct pressure does not control the bleeding from a limb, or the bleeding is catastrophic, apply a tourniquet above the wound to control bleeding (see sidebar, Using Tourniquets to Stem Bleeding).

6. Monitor for the development of shock (see Shock later in this chapter), record vital signs, and provide reassurance until EMS arrives.

The direct pressure needs to be applied over the bleeding point of the wound to be effective. Be aware that a large wound may have more than one active bleeding point.

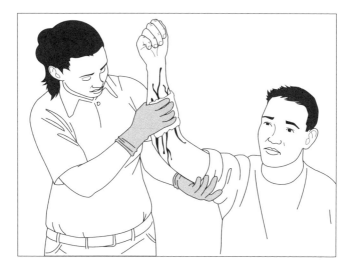

Apply continuous direct pressure to stop bleeding from a major wound.

Using Tourniquets to Stem Bleeding

Evidence has shown that tourniquets are an effective method of stopping major bleeding from a limb. They work by cutting off blood supply beyond the tourniquet, thereby stopping blood loss from the wound. Consider using a tourniquet for life-threatening bleeding from a limb that can't be controlled by firm direct pressure. Many large first aid kits now contain tourniquets. The tourniquet should be applied approximately three inches above the wound but not directly over a joint. Ensure you accurately record the time the tourniquet was applied and hand over this information to EMS.

Don't Remove Embedded Objects

If you notice a foreign object embedded in a wound, do not remove it. This could cause further bleeding or damage to the underlying tissues. Instead, apply pressure around the object in order to stop bleeding and seek urgent medical attention.

Amputation

An amputation occurs when a limb (or part of a limb) is severed from the body. Amputations can cause significant blood loss, and quick first aid treatment is important to stop severe bleeding and prevent shock. If possible, the amputated body part should be cooled to maximize the chances of surgical reattachment at the hospital. Amputations of fingers and thumbs are often caused by workplace or DIY injuries. Amputations of arms and legs are often seen following an explosion or other high-impact trauma such as a high-speed motor vehicle collision. Witnessing an amputation can be emotionally traumatizing for a rescuer, especially if there are multiple injured victims involved. The priority is to stop severe bleeding to buy the victim time before the arrival of EMS. Cooling the limb may increase the chances of it being surgically reattached at the hospital; however, it is important not to place the limb in direct contact with ice as this could damage it.

First Aid Treatment for an Amputation

1. Immediately call EMS.
2. Treat any severe bleeding (see Severe Bleeding earlier in this chapter) and monitor the victim for shock;

a tourniquet may be required to control bleeding from an amputated limb.

3. If possible, locate the amputated body part.

4. Wrap the amputated limb in a sterile dressing and a clean plastic bag.

5. Place the amputated limb in a container of ice-cold water if available.

The aim is to keep the amputated limb cool to increase the chances of surgical reattachment at the hospital. Do not place the amputated limb in direct contact with ice as this could damage the delicate tissues and blood vessels.

Puncture Wounds

A puncture wound occurs when a sharp object pierces the skin. A common example of a puncture wound is a victim stepping on a sharp object such as a nail. Animal bites are another relatively common cause of puncture wounds. We'll cover these in a different section of this pocket guide (see Animal Bites in Chapter 10). Puncture wounds may look minor, and there might not be much bleeding from the wound; however, they can cause serious complications such as infection and damage to underlying nerves and muscles. It is very difficult to assess how deep a puncture wound is, or what damage the object has caused underneath the wound. For this reason, all puncture wounds should be assessed by a medical professional. Many puncture wounds require an X-ray to ensure there are no fragments of the object still embedded in the wound. Surgical removal of any embedded objects may be required to reduce the risk of a serious infection developing and to allow the wound to heal properly.

First Aid Treatment for a Puncture Wound

1. Apply direct pressure to stop any bleeding.
2. If there is an object still embedded in the wound, do not remove it; instead, apply padding around the object and seek medical assistance.
3. If the wound has been bleeding heavily, monitor the victim for shock. Call EMS if you are concerned the victim is going into shock or you are unable to stem the bleeding.
4. Try to identify the object that caused the puncture wound.
5. Seek medical help; the victim may require antibiotic treatment to prevent a serious infection from developing.

Shock

You've probably heard the term *shock* used when people talk about an injured victim, but what exactly is shock, and why is it so important in first aid? Shock occurs when our body tissues do not receive an adequate supply of oxygen. Oxygen is vital to allow the tissues in our body to work properly. Without oxygen our cells cannot function and will start to die. This causes damage to the brain and other vital organs.

Severe blood loss is one cause of shock. This makes sense since there is less blood available to carry oxygen through the body to the cells. Shock is life-threatening and requires urgent medical intervention to replace the blood lost. There are other causes of shock besides blood loss. Major burn injuries can also cause shock as burns cause fluid to leak into the injury (see Major Burns later in this chapter), and therefore, there is less fluid flowing through the body for the rest of the cells. In addition, a victim suffering from anaphylaxis (a major allergic reaction) may also go into shock.

You need to be aware of the signs and symptoms of shock and constantly monitor a victim for the warning signs that may indicate shock. The shock we've described here is different from mental or psychological shock following a distressing event. People who witness a traumatic event are often described as being "in shock," but this is not the same as physical shock caused by excessive blood loss.

Signs and Symptoms of Shock

- Pale, cold, or clammy skin
- Increased pulse and respiratory rate
- Weak pulse that is difficult to find
- Vomiting
- Confusion
- Reduced level of consciousness (late sign)

First Aid Treatment for Shock

1. Immediately call EMS.

2. Find and treat the cause of the shock (for example, by stopping any serious bleeding).

3. Lay the victim down and elevate the legs six to twelve inches unless there is evidence of a leg or pelvic (hip) injury.

4. Keep the victim warm and do not give him anything to eat or drink.

5. Provide reassurance and monitor vital signs.

Your priority in first aid is to identify shock in a victim and stop it from worsening. You cannot replace the blood lost by a victim, but effective first aid can stop further blood loss and prevent the shock from worsening. In addition, rapid treatment of burns and anaphylaxis can also help prevent shock.

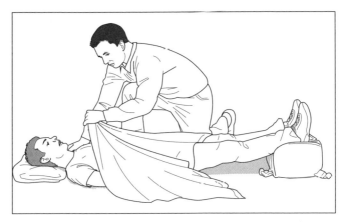

The correct first aid treatment position for a shock victim.

Fractures (Closed)

Fractures (or broken bones) are common injuries among children and adults, and many of us will break at least one bone in our lifetime. A fracture occurs when excessive force is applied to a bone resulting in the bone breaking. Simple trips and falls cause the majority of fractures, especially to the arm and wrist. Athletics and adventure sports are common causes of broken legs and ankles. Sometimes it can be difficult to tell the difference between a fracture and a soft-tissue injury (sprain or strain); there have been many cases of people walking around for several days on a broken ankle before seeking help! An X-ray is required to tell if a bone is broken, so always seek medical attention if you are concerned that a victim may have fractured a bone.

Let's look at the main types of fractures you might encounter.

A closed fracture occurs when a bone is broken but does not cause a break in the skin. The majority of fractures are closed. If the bone does cut through the skin, this is known as an open fracture. Any wound overlying a fracture should be suspected to be caused by an open fracture. We'll take a closer look at open fractures in the next section.

Complicated fractures occur when the broken bone damages blood vessels or nerves near the fracture site. These fractures require urgent specialist medical treatment to reduce the risk of long-term complications such as permanent nerve damage. Fractures may occur alongside a dislocation (for example, a dislocated shoulder can also be broken). We'll discuss dislocations in another section.

Fractures can be very painful for a victim, especially if the limb is badly broken. Your main aim in first aid is to prevent excessive movement of the fracture to reduce pain and any internal bleeding. All fracture victims require an X-ray and assessment by a medical professional. Some fractures may require realignment in the hospital, and in some cases surgery to fix the broken bone.

Medical Terminology

The medical term for *broken bone* is *fracture*. These two terms mean the same thing.

Signs and Symptoms of a Fracture

These signs and symptoms can be remembered by using the acronym PLASTIC. It is easier to assess for angulation or irregularity in a limb by comparing the suspected fracture to the other unaffected side.

- **P**ain
- **L**oss of movement
- **A**ngulation (abnormal bend or curve) of the limb
- **S**welling
- **T**enderness
- **I**rregularity
- **C**repitus (a cracking or grating sound)

First Aid Treatment for a Fracture

1. Treat any severe bleeding (see Severe Bleeding earlier in this chapter).

2. Stabilize the injury to prevent movement of the fracture.

3. If the fracture is open, apply a sterile dressing over the wound to reduce the risk of infection.

4. Check for signs of circulation beyond the fracture (see sidebar, Checking for Circulation); if circulation beyond the injury appears to be damaged, seek urgent medical assistance.

5. Monitor the victim for shock and record vital signs (see sidebar, Watch Out for Shock).

6. Seek medical assistance or call EMS.

Watch Out for Shock

A fracture of a large bone, such as the femur or pelvis, can cause significant internal bleeding. The victim may lose so much blood that she starts to go into shock (see Shock earlier in this chapter). Always monitor a victim with a suspected major fracture for shock.

Checking for Circulation

A complicated fracture may damage the circulation in a limb. This is an emergency and could lead to permanent paralysis or, at worst, require amputation. Signs of compromised circulation include the limb turning pale or blue or feeling cold to the touch. The victim may complain of numbness in the limb and be unable to move the affected area.

First Aid Treatment for a Fractured Arm

1. Follow the general first aid steps for a fracture (see earlier section in this chapter).

2. Pad around the injury and support above and below the fracture using your hands.

3. Place the affected arm in an arm sling (see Appendix A: First Aid Techniques).

4. If no sling is available, ask the victim to support the arm in the most comfortable position; take caution to avoid any excessive movement of the injured arm.

5. Seek medical attention; the victim will require an X-ray to assess the injury and decide on the correct ongoing treatment.

First Aid Treatment for a Fractured Leg

1. Follow the general first aid steps for a fracture (see earlier section in this chapter).

2. Pad around the injury and support above and below the fracture using your hands or by applying a splint if trained.

3. Call EMS.

4. Do not allow the victim to walk or put weight on the injury.

5. Do not attempt to realign or straighten the leg.

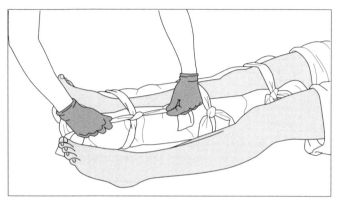

For a fractured leg, pad around the injury.

Fractures (Open)

Open fractures occur when there is a wound caused by a broken bone piercing the skin.

Open fractures are more severe than closed fractures as there is a significant risk of infection in the exposed bone; this can lead to widespread infection or even the loss of a limb. Thankfully, open fractures are relatively rare as they require a lot of force to occur. However, that a fracture is open sometimes can go unnoticed; the bone may not always be visible in the wound. After an injury the muscles around a fracture go into spasm, and this can pull the exposed bone back underneath the skin. For this reason, you should assume any wound overlying a fracture is caused by an open fracture until proven otherwise.

Your main aim in first aid when dealing with an open fracture is to control any life-threatening bleeding and reduce the risk of infection. Place a sterile dressing over the wound or exposed bone as soon as possible to reduce the risk of the bone becoming contaminated. Open fractures are painful, and the victim is likely to be very distressed with the injury, so remain calm and provide reassurance until medical help arrives. All open fractures normally require surgery to thoroughly clean the injury and the administration of strong antibiotics to prevent a severe bone infection from developing.

Medical Terminology

The medical term for an open fracture is *compound fracture*.

First Aid Treatment for an Open Fracture

1. Call EMS.

2. Treat any severe bleeding (see Severe Bleeding earlier in this chapter); an open fracture can cause severe bleeding if the broken bone has damaged a large blood vessel.

3. Stabilize the injury to prevent movement of the fracture; further movement could worsen any bleeding.

4. Apply a sterile dressing over the wound to reduce the risk of infection.

5. Monitor the victim for shock (see sidebar, Watch Out for Shock) and record vital signs until EMS arrives.

Dislocations

A dislocation occurs when a bone moves out of the correct position at a joint. These injuries can be very painful, as anyone who has experienced a dislocated joint will know! Common sites for dislocations include the shoulder, wrist, and fingers. A common cause of a dislocated joint is excessive force being applied to the joint (for example, following a fall). A dislocation injury may be accompanied by a fracture, and it is difficult to assess for a fracture. Therefore, most victims require an X-ray before attempting to reduce the bone back into the joint. It is important that you do not attempt to relocate, or reduce, a dislocated joint; the victim requires assessment by a medical professional. Otherwise, you risk causing further permanent damage to the bone, nerves, or blood vessels. Your main aim is to support the joint in the position found and prevent further movement of the injured area.

A dislocation injury may cause damage to the ligaments that support a joint. This can make the joint unstable and the victim more prone to recurrent dislocations. Physical therapy or, in some cases, surgery may be required to fix and strengthen the ligaments to prevent dislocations from occurring. A victim who has suffered a dislocation injury should seek advice from a medical professional or physiotherapist before returning to any athletic activity, especially contact sports.

Signs and Symptoms of a Dislocation

The signs and symptoms of a dislocation are similar to those of a fracture:

- Pain
- Loss of movement
- Angulation of the limb
- Swelling
- Tenderness
- Irregularity
- Crepitus (a cracking or grating sound)

The abnormal angulation of a limb may be more prominent in a dislocation injury. You should compare the affected limb with the unaffected side of the body to assess for angulation and irregularity.

First Aid Treatment for a Dislocated Joint

1. Support the limb in the position found; do not attempt to reduce the dislocation.

2. Apply padding around the injury.

3. Check for signs of circulation beyond the injury (see sidebar, Checking for Circulation).

4. If the victim has dislocated his shoulder, elbow, or wrist, then an arm sling may be useful to support the injury (see Appendix A: First Aid Techniques).

5. Seek medical assistance or call EMS.

Shoulder Dislocation Following a Seizure

A victim having a major seizure is at risk of a shoulder dislocation due to excessive muscle contractions. Do not attempt to restrain a victim having a seizure in order to prevent a dislocation. You are likely to cause injury to yourself or the victim and worsen the situation.

Crush Injuries

Major crush injuries are life-threatening situations and will require early specialist help to safely extricate and treat the victim. A major crush injury occurs when a large part of the body (for example, the chest) is crushed. An example of this is a victim trapped underneath a car following a motor vehicle collision. These victims often have multiple injuries and require advanced medical help at the scene of the incident, so never delay in calling for EMS. Minor crush injuries, such as fingers or toes, often occur in the workplace or when performing projects at home. A crush injury can be complicated by bleeding or a fracture of the bones underneath the skin.

Be aware that victims of major crush injuries are at risk of developing crush injury syndrome. This syndrome occurs when a major crush injury causes the buildup of toxins in the damaged tissue. When the object causing the crush is removed, and pressure on the injury is released, these toxins spread through the body and can cause fatal heart abnormalities and kidney damage. As a result, a major crush injury victim can quickly deteriorate after the crushing object has been removed.

First Aid Treatment for a Major Crush Injury

1. Ensure the scene is safe for you to approach.
2. Call EMS.
3. If safe to do so, release the pressure on the crush injury victim as soon as possible.
4. Look for and treat any severe bleeding found (see Severe Bleeding earlier in this chapter).
5. Monitor for shock (see Shock earlier in this chapter), monitor vital signs, and provide reassurance until the arrival of EMS.

If the victim has been trapped for a long time, releasing pressure may lead to the development of crush injury syndrome and the victim may quickly deteriorate. If a victim has been trapped for a prolonged period, communicate with the EMS operator and seek expert advice.

Head Injuries

Head injuries can range from minor bumps to life-threatening head trauma. Our brains are made up of a delicate network of cells and pathways that enable us to think and control our bodies. The skull is responsible for protecting our brain from knocks and bumps. Minor head injuries often cause concussions. What exactly does this term mean?

A concussion occurs when the brain is shaken in the skull, causing a temporary disturbance in brain functioning. However, any head injury carries the risk of bleeding or swelling inside the brain. This situation is life-threatening; because the skull is a fixed box, it does not allow the brain to bulge outward or swell. Therefore, any swelling or bleeding in the brain will rapidly increase the pressure inside the skull and cause the delicate brain cells and networks to be compressed. This situation can develop rapidly and lead to life-threatening and life-changing brain damage. The symptoms of a severe head injury may be delayed by several hours after the initial injury as the pressure in the skull can take time to build up. As a result, all head injury victims should be evaluated by a trained medical professional.

In addition to injuries to the brain, the bones of the skull can be fractured following a direct blow to the head. Skull fractures can bleed significantly, and they expose the delicate brain tissue to the outside environment, so there is a risk of infection. These injuries often require the victim to undergo surgery to fix the fracture and strong antibiotics to prevent brain infection.

Any victim with a serious head injury is presumed to have a neck injury (see Neck and Back Injuries later in this chapter) until evaluated by a medical professional. The head is connected to the body via the spine; therefore, blows to the head can put stress on the neck and risk causing a spinal injury.

Signs and Symptoms of Concussion

- A brief loss of consciousness
- Headache
- Memory loss of the incident
- Nausea
- Dizziness
- Visual disturbance (for example, blurred or double vision)

Signs and Symptoms of a Life-Threatening Head Injury

- A temporary improvement in consciousness, followed by decreasing responsiveness
- Vomiting
- One pupil larger than the other
- Evidence of a skull fracture or severe bleeding from a head wound

- Seizures
- Blood or fluid leaking from the nose or ears
- Evidence of a skull fracture
- Severe memory loss of events before or after the head injury

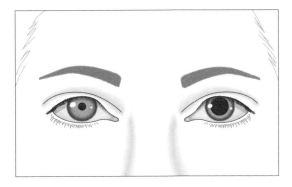

A large pupil in one eye following a head injury is a sign of a life-threatening injury.

First Aid Treatment for a Major Head Injury

1. Call EMS.

2. Treat any severe bleeding from the head by applying direct pressure.

3. Support the victim's head and neck in the position found; avoid excessive movement of the victim.

4. Monitor vital signs and level of consciousness (see sidebar, Monitoring Level of Consciousness Using AVPU).

5. If the victim becomes unconscious and her airway is blocked, she will need to be carefully turned into the recovery position to protect the airway (see The Recovery Position in Chapter 3).

6. Be prepared to perform CPR if the victim stops breathing normally (see Cardiopulmonary Resuscitation (CPR) in Chapter 3).

Monitoring Level of Consciousness Using AVPU

Following a head injury, a victim may have a reduced level of consciousness. To assess this, you can use the AVPU scale:

- **A**lert: The victim is alert and conversing with you
- **V**oice: The victim only responds to verbal instructions
- **P**ain: The victim only responds to a pain stimulus (for example, pinching the top of the shoulder)
- **U**nconscious: The victim does not respond to a verbal or painful stimulus

Blood-Thinning Medication

Some people take blood-thinning (anticoagulant) medication for heart conditions or following a blood clot. Examples of these medications include warfarin (Coumadin), rivaroxaban, apixaban, and dabigatran. Any victim who has had a head injury, however minor, while taking blood-thinning medication must seek urgent medical help, as he may require a scan of his brain to check for internal bleeding.

Neck and Back Injuries

The spine is the major structure in the neck and back, but what exactly makes up our spines? Our spines are composed of individual bones that form a tunnel stretching from the top of the neck to the lower back. Through this tunnel runs the spinal cord, a complex network of nerves and cells, which sends signals to and from the brain. The spinal cord is responsible for transmitting sensory information to the brain (for example, the sensation of pain) and for conveying commands from the brain to the muscles (for example, to move your arm). As well as carrying the spinal cord, the bones of the spine support the body and provide an attachment for many muscles that give us flexibility and strength.

Excessive force applied to the back or neck can fracture the bones that make up the spine and cause permanent damage to the spinal cord. This force could be from a direct blow or a trauma situation such as a fall from height or high-speed motor vehicle collision (see sidebar, When to Suspect a Neck or Back Injury).

Spinal cord injury can cause permanent paralysis of limbs and a loss of sensation. This is a devastating, life-changing injury for the victim and often requires a long period of rehabilitation.

How can you help a victim with a suspected neck or back injury? The key is to minimize any movement of the victim following the injury. Further movement following an injury to the spine can cause more damage to the spinal cord and worsen the injury. Therefore, your priority is to keep the victim as still as possible before the arrival of EMS. Remember, preventing worsening of the victim's condition is one of the key aims in any first aid situation.

Medical Terminology

The individual bones that make up the spine are called *vertebrae*.

When to Suspect a Neck or Back Injury

You should suspect that a victim may have sustained a neck or back injury in the following situations:

- Fall from height
- High-speed motor vehicle collision
- Head injury with reduced level of consciousness
- Direct blow to the neck or back
- Head injury from diving into a shallow pool

- Horseback-riding accident (for example, being thrown from a horse)
- Multiple traumatic injuries
- An injured victim under the influence of alcohol or drugs

Signs and Symptoms of a Neck or Back Injury

- Neck or back pain
- Evidence of a serious head injury
- Loss of movement of arms or legs
- Altered sensation in arms or legs (numbness, burning, or tingling sensations)
- Loss of control of bladder or bowels

First Aid Treatment for a Neck or Back Injury (Victim Is Awake)

If the victim is awake, then you should:

1. Call EMS.

2. Keep the victim supported in the position found; avoid any movement of the head, neck, or back.

3. Kneel or lie down above the victim's head and place your hands on both sides of his head to keep the neck still; do not attempt to realign the neck.

4. If available, place rolled-up blankets or towels on either side of the head to minimize movement of the neck.

5. Monitor vital signs and level of consciousness until EMS arrives.

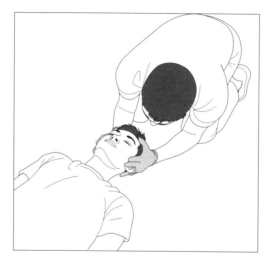

Support a victim's neck by holding the head in the position found.

First Aid Treatment for a Neck or Back Injury (Victim Is Unresponsive)

If the victim is unresponsive, then you should follow the DR ABC action plan described in Chapter 3 but with some modifications. Check that the situation is safe to approach and the victim is unresponsive. Ensure EMS has been called. Then:

1. Open the airway using the jaw thrust technique:

   a. Kneel above the victim's head.

   b. Place your hands on each side of his head with your thumbs over his cheekbones.

   c. Using your fingers, lift the jaw forward but do not tilt the head backward.

2. Check for the presence of normal breathing.

3. If the victim is not breathing, immediately update EMS and commence CPR (see Cardiopulmonary Resuscitation (CPR) in Chapter 3).

4. If the victim is breathing normally, try to support him in the position found and maintain his airway with a jaw thrust.

5. If the victim is breathing normally, but he is vomiting or his airway is obstructed, then he will need to be turned into the recovery position to protect his airway (see sidebar, Using the Recovery Position).

Using the Recovery Position

A victim with a suspected neck or back injury should be moved as little as possible in order to protect his spine. Ideally, he should be left in the position he is found in. However, if the victim is on his back and you are unable to keep his airway open using a jaw thrust (for example, because he is vomiting), then he is at risk of choking. You will need to carefully turn the victim onto his side, ideally with one person supporting the head and neck in line with the rest of the body, using the technique described in Chapter 3. If more helpers are available, they can support the back and neck as the victim rolls over to minimize movement of the spine.

Major Burns

More than a million Americans each year require medical attention due to burn injuries. Major burn injuries can be life-threatening and life-changing because of the risk of permanent scarring. You can really make a difference to a burn injury victim by providing early effective first aid treatment for the burn and by calling for EMS early.

Why is early first aid treatment vital for burn injury victims? The burning process continues even after the cause of the burn has been removed. This causes further damage to the skin and underlying tissues. Cooling with running water will remove heat from the burn and prevent further damage from occurring. Burns that are cooled quickly will heal faster and with fewer complications such as long-term scarring. When cooling a burn, you need to be aware of the risk of hypothermia setting in, especially in children with major burns. Try to keep a victim warm while cooling the affected area (see sidebar, Cool the Burn, Warm the Victim).

Burn injuries can be classified into three different depths (see sidebar, Burn Injury Depths). Most burns are due to contact with a hot surface or liquid, which causes damage to the skin and underlying tissues. However, there are other causes of burns, including chemicals and the sun. We'll cover these types of burns in a different part of this pocket guide.

You need to watch out for shock in a burn victim. Major burns cause significant loss of fluid through the damaged skin. This can cause shock (see Shock earlier in this chapter). Always monitor a major burn victim for signs and symptoms of shock.

Burn Injury Depths

Burn injuries can be broadly divided into three different depths:

- Superficial (first degree): damage to the top layer of skin cells
- Partial (second degree): blistering of the skin

■ Full thickness (third degree): damage to deep muscle and soft tissues

You may find a burn injury has areas of different depths. For example, a severe burn may be third degree in the center with areas of second- and first-degree burns surrounding it.

First Aid Treatment for Major Burns

1. Call EMS.
2. Immediately cool the burned area with cool running water for a minimum of twenty minutes.
3. Cover the burn loosely with a non-fluffy sterile dressing. Clean plastic wrap can be used if no sterile dressings are available.
4. If the burn is affecting a limb, remove any rings, watches, or straps near the burned area.
5. Monitor the victim for hypothermia (see sidebar, Cool the Burn, Warm the Victim).

Major burn injuries can be life-threatening, especially in children and the elderly. Always call EMS for a major burn victim. In addition, infection is a common complication following burns, and these injuries need careful assessment and management by a specialist burn center.

Common Burn Injury Myths

There are many myths regarding the first aid treatment of burns. Major burns need to be quickly cooled with running water in order to stop the burning process.

■ Do not apply toothpaste or butter to a burn. This will not cool the burn adequately. The best method to cool a major burn is to run cold water over it.
■ Do not burst blisters as this will increase the risk of infection.
■ Do not remove clothing stuck to burned skin. This can cause further damage to the skin.

Cool the Burn, Warm the Victim

Major burns require rapid cooling in order to stop the burning process. If a victim has burns covering large areas of her body, this cooling process may lead to the body's temperature dropping, resulting in hypothermia. You need to take steps to avoid hypothermia by monitoring the victim and attempting to keep her warm, while cooling the burn. For example, blankets can be used to cover non-burned areas. It is important to prevent hypothermia, since low body temperature can cause further complications for victims with major burns.

Chemical Burns

Strong chemicals can cause burns to the skin and underlying tissues. Although they are less common than heat burns, chemical burns can cause major injury to a victim and may be associated with the production of toxic fumes. You must always consider your own safety before entering a potentially hazardous situation involving chemicals. Remember, you are the most important person in any emergency situation!

Chemical burns may occur in the workplace due to strong chemicals used in manufacturing or other industrial tasks. Employers have a responsibility for the health and safety of their employees, and adequate emergency equipment should be available to deal with a chemical incident should it occur. In the home, some strong domestic cleaning products (for example, oven or drain cleaners) can also cause chemical burns. These products should come with clear warning signs and instructions on how to treat accidental poisoning or injury. Children are at risk of sustaining accidental chemical burns from household products as they may be attracted by the bright colors or strong smells of the products.

Your main aim in first aid is to dilute the chemical responsible for causing the burn to reduce ongoing burning. This will require lots of running water (for example, from a garden hose).

The waste runoff water should be treated as potentially contaminated with chemicals. Make sure the runoff water is directed away from you and the victim.

First Aid Treatment for Chemical Burns

1. Ensure the scene is safe for you to approach; be aware of the risk of toxic fumes from chemicals.

2. Immediately call EMS, and tell the emergency operator that the victim has come into contact with dangerous chemicals.

3. Flood the burned area with running water for at least twenty minutes, ensuring the runoff wastewater is directed away from the victim and you.

4. Remove contaminated clothing if safe to do so.

5. Try to identify the substance that caused the burn and hand over this information to EMS when they arrive.

When Not to Use Water

Chemical burns caused by contact with elemental metals (magnesium, lithium, sodium, potassium, and phosphorus) or dry lime should not be flooded with water as contact with water will cause a chemical reaction on the victim's skin. If a powder is visible on the skin, it should be brushed off as quickly as possible.

Chemical Burns to the Eye

Strong chemicals splashing into the eye can cause permanent damage to the eye and loss of sight. If a victim has chemicals in his eye, irrigate the eye for at least twenty minutes (see Appendix A: First Aid Techniques) and seek urgent medical attention. Do not attempt to neutralize the chemical by putting other substances into the eye; this could cause further harm.

Chapter Seven
MEDICAL EMERGENCIES

BEING ABLE TO SPOT THE WARNING SIGNS of a serious medical emergency is an important skill in first aid. The victim may not always appreciate the seriousness of the symptoms she is experiencing, so it is your role to recognize the important warning signs and summon early medical help. You can also make a difference and potentially save a life by administering early treatment (for example, by offering an aspirin to a heart attack victim). You also need to know what not to do. Unfortunately, there are many myths circulating about treating medical conditions such as seizures (fits). Some of these incorrect beliefs could make the situation much worse and cause harm to the victim. In this chapter, we'll guide you through some of the most important medical emergencies and how to recognize them and start early treatment; we'll also debunk some of the most common first aid myths. Let's start by looking at heart attacks, one of the most serious medical emergencies you may encounter.

Heart Attack

The heart is a muscular pump responsible for moving blood through the body. Our hearts need an excellent blood supply to provide enough oxygen to keep the heart muscle pumping effectively. A heart attack occurs when the blood supply to the heart is interrupted, leading to part of the heart muscle being injured or dying. This is different from cardiac arrest (see sidebar, Heart Attack versus Cardiac Arrest).

Why does a heart attack happen? The blood vessels that supply the heart are called the coronary arteries. As we age, our coronary arteries can become lined with plaque, which contains cholesterol and other fatty substances that build up in the wall of the artery. Lifestyle factors including smoking, obesity, and an unhealthy diet all accelerate this process.

Over time, the fatty buildup in the lining of the artery increases. Eventually, this fatty buildup can rupture, resulting in the formation of a blood clot. This blood clot blocks the artery and stops blood from flowing to the vital heart muscle. The heart muscle becomes starved of oxygen and starts to die. This causes the victim to experience the common signs and symptoms of a heart attack.

A heart attack requires emergency medical treatment to unblock the artery and restore blood flow to the affected muscle.

You must not delay in calling EMS if you suspect a victim is having a heart attack. The quicker the blockage in the artery is cleared, the more likely it is that the heart muscle will make a complete recovery.

Medical Terminology

The medical term for a heart attack is *myocardial infarction (MI)*. The term *myocardial* refers to the heart muscle, and *infarction* means the death of tissue due to lack of oxygen.

Heart Attack versus Cardiac Arrest

The terms *heart attack* and *cardiac arrest* are commonly confused, especially in the media. A heart attack is a medical condition caused by a blockage of a blood vessel supplying the heart. Cardiac arrest occurs when the heart stops pumping blood through the body, so the victim loses consciousness and stops breathing. A heart attack may cause cardiac arrest, but there are many other causes of cardiac arrest.

Signs and Symptoms of a Heart Attack

- Chest pain that may radiate to the jaw, back, arms, or stomach
- Shortness of breath
- Excessive sweating

- Increased pulse and respiratory rate
- Pale skin
- Nausea and/or vomiting

The pain from a heart attack can vary. The classic description is central crushing chest pain. However, any sensation of pain or pressure in the chest should be considered as coming from the heart until proven otherwise.

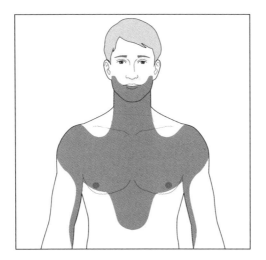

The pain from a heart attack can spread into the jaw, arms, and stomach.

Watch Out for Silent Heart Attacks

Some heart attacks may not present with the typical symptoms of chest pain radiating to the arm. In rare cases, a victim may have no pain at all. Women and people with diabetes are more likely to experience these "silent" heart attacks. Victims who have a silent heart attack may only have mild pain mistaken for heartburn or a pulled muscle. In some cases, the victim has no symptoms at all.

First Aid Treatment for a Heart Attack

If you suspect a victim may be having a heart attack, you should:

1. Immediately call EMS.

2. Place the victim in a comfortable position and loosen any tight clothing.

3. Offer to administer a regular strength (325 mg) aspirin tablet if appropriate (see sidebar, Administering Aspirin to a Heart Attack Victim).

4. Be prepared to perform cardiopulmonary resuscitation (CPR) if the victim loses consciousness and stops breathing (see Cardiopulmonary Resuscitation (CPR) in Chapter 3).

5. Provide reassurance and monitor vital signs until emergency medical help arrives.

Administering Aspirin to a Heart Attack Victim

Early administration of aspirin has been shown to improve the chances of survival from a heart attack. Aspirin helps break down the clot in the blocked blood vessel.

- The aspirin tablet should be chewed and swallowed by the victim.
- Do not administer aspirin if the victim has a known aspirin allergy or a history of recent bleeding.

If you are concerned about administering aspirin, seek advice from EMS over the telephone or await the arrival of expert medical help. Most first aid kits contain emergency aspirin for use in a heart attack situation.

Stroke (Brain Attack)

Our brain cells require a constant supply of oxygen and nutrients to function effectively. A stroke occurs when the blood supply to the brain is interrupted. This interruption in blood supply causes brain cells to die and can result in permanent brain damage. Stroke victims require emergency medical treatment to restore blood flow to the damaged brain tissue. There are two types of stroke; let's take a look at these in more detail.

The most common type of stroke is caused by a blood clot in the blood vessels supplying the brain. The blood clot blocks the vessel, leading to the brain cells being starved of oxygen and nutrients, eventually causing cell death. This is known as an ischemic stroke.

The second type of stroke is caused by a bleed into the brain from a ruptured blood vessel, leading to brain swelling and cell death. This type of stroke is known as a hemorrhagic stroke. Hemorrhagic strokes are much less common than ischemic strokes and are more common in people who take blood-thinning medication.

Medical Terminology

The medical term for a stroke is *cerebrovascular event (CVE)* or *cerebrovascular accident (CVA)*. The medical term *hemorrhagic* refers to bleeding.

The treatment for an ischemic stroke is similar to the treatment for a heart attack. The affected blood vessel needs to be unblocked to restore blood flow to the damaged brain tissue. The faster this happens, the more likely the brain cells are to recover and the less likely there will be permanent brain damage. Victims need to have the blood flow restored within three hours to save vital brain tissue and have the best chance of making a good recovery. Therefore, you must not delay in calling EMS if you suspect a victim is having a stroke.

Strokes are now also known as brain attacks, which emphasizes the importance of calling for help early, as you do when you are dealing with a suspected heart attack.

Signs and Symptoms of a Stroke

- Facial droop on one side
- Loss of power down one side of the body
- Slurred speech
- Sudden loss of vision
- Dizziness
- Reduced level of consciousness
- Seizures

The most common symptoms of a stroke can be remembered by using the acronym FAST.

- **F**ace: Is there any facial droop?
- **A**rms: Can the victim raise both arms?
- **S**peech: Is there any slurred speech?
- **T**ime: Time to call EMS if any one of these symptoms is present.

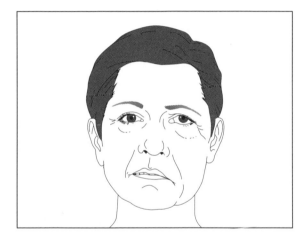

A stroke victim may have a facial droop on one side.

First Aid Treatment for a Stroke

If you suspect a victim may be having a stroke, you should:

1. Immediately call EMS.

2. Place the victim in a comfortable position.

3. Record the time of onset of the symptoms and inform EMS.

4. Provide reassurance and monitor vital signs until emergency medical help arrives.

5. Do not give the victim anything to eat or drink, as there is a risk of choking.

Never administer aspirin to a stroke victim. There is no way in first aid to distinguish between a stroke caused by a bleed (hemorrhagic) or one caused by a clot (ischemic). Administering aspirin will worsen a stroke caused by a bleeding blood vessel.

Watch Out for Mini-Strokes

A mini-stroke occurs when the symptoms of a stroke resolve within twenty-four hours with no medical treatment. The medical term for this is *transient ischemic attack (TIA)*. A mini-stroke often occurs before a major stroke, so a TIA should be treated as a serious warning sign. You cannot distinguish a mini-stroke from a regular stroke; therefore, always call EMS if a victim shows any of the signs and symptoms of a stroke. Do not wait to see if the symptoms resolve on their own before seeking medical assistance.

Asthma

Most of us know someone who is living with asthma. Asthma is a common long-term condition that affects the small air passages in the lungs. During an asthma attack, these small air passages become swollen and blocked with phlegm. This narrows the air passages and restricts air flow through the lungs, which causes the victim to experience difficulty in breathing and often creates a characteristic wheezing noise. Wheezing is a high-pitched whistling noise caused by air trying to flow through the swollen air passages. Why does this swelling happen?

People often develop asthma in childhood. The air passages become sensitive to inhaled particles and environmental changes. These are known as asthma triggers. Common triggers include pollen, air pollution, changes in air temperature, and exercise. When the body comes into contact with a trigger, it responds by releasing chemicals into the air passages, which cause swelling and the production of excessive mucus (phlegm). This causes the victim to experience the signs and symptoms of an asthma attack.

Despite modern medical advances, asthma can still be life-threatening, and there are still deaths every year from acute asthma attacks. A victim having an asthma attack can get worse very quickly, so you should always seek medical advice if you are concerned about his breathing.

Signs and Symptoms of an Asthma Attack

- Difficulty in breathing
- A wheezing sound
- A sensation of chest tightness
- Persistent coughing
- Increased respiratory and pulse rate

During severe attacks, the victim may become exhausted and have a decreased level of consciousness. His skin may also turn pale and have a blue tinge around the mouth, ears, or fingernails. These features indicate life-threatening asthma, and emergency medical help is urgently required.

First Aid Treatment for an Asthma Attack

If you suspect a victim is having an asthma attack you should:

1. Assist the victim in using his inhaled asthma medication.

2. Provide reassurance and monitor vital signs.

3. Immediately call for EMS if:

   a. There is no improvement in symptoms after using his inhaler.

   b. The victim is not carrying any medication.

   c. You are worried about the severity of the asthma attack.

Do not delay in calling EMS if you are concerned about a victim with asthma. Life-threatening asthma can develop over minutes and requires immediate emergency medical treatment. If in doubt, call for professional medical help.

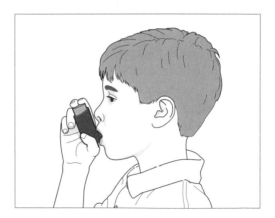

An asthma inhaler is used to relieve the symptoms of an asthma attack.

Asthma Inhalers

Patients with asthma should carry a "reliever" inhaler. This inhaler contains medication (salbutamol) to combat the swelling during an asthma attack and helps to improve breathing. Patients with asthma should be trained by a medical professional in how to use their inhalers effectively.

Anaphylaxis (Severe Allergic Reaction)

Anaphylaxis is a severe, life-threatening, allergic reaction affecting the entire body. Many of us know someone at risk of anaphylaxis, as the condition is becoming more common. Anaphylaxis occurs when the body becomes overly sensitive to a certain trigger. Common triggers of anaphylaxis include food products (nuts, shellfish, fish); insect venom (bees, wasps, ants); medications (antibiotics); and latex. How do these substances cause anaphylaxis?

When the body comes into contact with a trigger, it reacts by releasing large amounts of histamine. In small quantities, histamine is responsible for causing the signs of a mild allergic reaction such as itching or minor swelling. However, when the body releases a massive amount of histamine, it causes a whole body reaction. This severe reaction is life-threatening as it causes swelling of the throat and can rapidly obstruct breathing.

The initial emergency treatment of anaphylaxis involves the rapid administration of the drug epinephrine. Epinephrine works to combat the effects of the histamine and reduces the life-threatening swelling. Because anaphylaxis can be fatal in minutes, patients are prescribed epinephrine auto-injector devices for self-administration before the arrival of emergency medical help. Your role is to summon emergency medical assistance and assist the victim in using her auto-injector device.

Signs and Symptoms of Anaphylaxis

- Hives (red itchy bumps appearing on the skin)
- Swelling of the face, tongue, or throat
- Difficulty in breathing
- Loss of consciousness
- Increased pulse and respiratory rate
- Vomiting
- Abdominal pain

The signs and symptoms of anaphylaxis can develop rapidly over minutes following contact with the trigger.

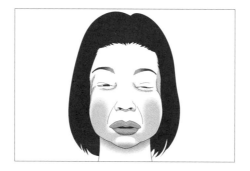

Swelling of the face and a red itchy rash are common signs of anaphylaxis.

First Aid Treatment for Anaphylaxis

1. Immediately call EMS.

2. If possible, remove the trigger of the anaphylaxis episode.

3. Assist the person in using her prescribed epinephrine auto-injector (see following sidebar).

4. Lay the victim down unless she is having significant breathing problems.

5. Be prepared to perform cardiopulmonary resuscitation (CPR) if the victim loses consciousness and stops breathing (see Cardiopulmonary Resuscitation (CPR) in Chapter 3).

6. Provide reassurance and monitor vital signs until emergency medical help arrives.

Rapid use of an auto-injector may resolve the victim's symptoms. However, medical help must still be sought, as there is a risk of a second delayed reaction.

Epinephrine Auto-Injectors

People with a known severe allergy should carry an epinephrine auto-injector at all times. These devices are designed to inject epinephrine into the thigh muscle during an anaphylaxis episode. There are a variety of brand names, but the most common brand is EpiPen. Auto-injectors have clear instructions on how to use them on the packaging or printed on the devices themselves.

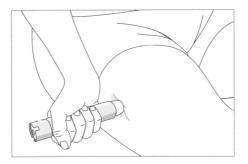

An epinephrine auto-injector is administered in the side of the thigh to treat life-threatening anaphylaxis.

Meningitis

Meningitis is a serious infection that affects the brain and spinal cord. The main risk from meningitis is that the infection can spread to the bloodstream and be fatal within hours. Why does meningitis occur? Our brains and spinal cords are covered by layers of protective membranes known as meninges. These membranes protect the delicate cells that make up the brain and spinal cord. A variety of bacteria and viruses can infect the meninges and cause inflammation; this is called meningitis. The infection can then spread to the victim's bloodstream and cause blood poisoning (septicemia). This causes the characteristic rash associated with meningitis, which doesn't go away when it is pressed on. Septicemia is life-threatening and requires urgent treatment in the hospital to combat the infection.

Anyone is at risk of catching meningitis. However, children and young people are the most vulnerable. Babies under the age of one year have the highest risk of developing meningitis. Vaccinations play an important role in reducing the risk of meningitis in babies and children, and the number of cases of meningitis has been decreasing. However, vaccinations do not protect against every virus that can cause meningitis. The treatment of meningitis and septicemia involves the rapid administration of strong antibiotics to combat the infection. Delays in administering antibiotics can be fatal; therefore, if you suspect meningitis, do not delay in calling for emergency medical help.

If you come into close contact with a victim who may be suffering from meningitis, then you should also seek medical assistance. In some cases, doctors will prescribe antibiotics to protect you from developing the disease.

Medical Terminology

When an infection spreads to the bloodstream, this is known as *septicemia*.

Signs and Symptoms of Meningitis

- Headache
- High temperature (fever)
- Neck stiffness
- Sensitivity to light (photophobia)
- Vomiting
- Lethargy
- Loss of appetite
- Reduced level of consciousness
- Seizures

As the infection spreads to the bloodstream, victims may become drowsy or confused or have a seizure. There may be elevated pulse and respiratory rates. In late stages, a rash may develop, which does not go away when it is pressed on. This is called a non-blanching rash and is a sign of severe blood poisoning (septicemia). Blood poisoning does not always cause a rash, so you must not wait for a rash to develop before calling for help (see sidebar, Don't Wait for a Rash).

First Aid Treatment for Meningitis

1. Immediately call EMS if you are concerned about the possibility of meningitis.

2. Provide reassurance and monitor vital signs until emergency medical help arrives.

There is no effective first aid treatment for meningitis. The victim will require early advanced medical care. Your role is to spot the warning signs that could indicate meningitis and seek early medical help without delay.

Don't Wait for a Rash

You must not wait for the development of a rash before calling for medical help. Some patients with severe blood poisoning may not develop a rash at all. If a rash does develop, the tumbler test can be used to determine whether the rash is suggestive of blood poisoning. If the rash does not disappear when a glass tumbler is rolled over it, this indicates blood poisoning.

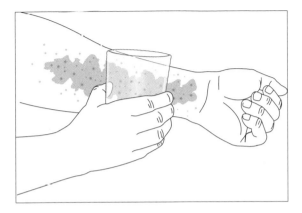

The tumbler test for a meningitis rash.

Seizures

A seizure occurs due to disorganized and excessive electrical activity in the brain. Our brain cells communicate using coordinated electrical activity among cells. When this activity becomes disrupted, a seizure results. There are two broad categories of seizure, generalized and focal. Let's look at these in more detail.

Generalized seizures are caused by abnormal electrical activity in the entire brain. These seizures may cause convulsions in which

the victim falls to the floor and has uncontrollable muscle movements. Victims may be unconscious during a generalized seizure.

In contrast, focal seizures affect only part of the brain. They
cause more limited symptoms than generalized seizures, and the
victim may be aware of the seizure occurring.

People with epilepsy may experience a particular sensation
or feeling before the start of a seizure. Typical examples include
an unusual smell or visual hallucination. This is known as an aura
and indicates a seizure may be about to occur.

Although seizures can appear distressing, short seizures that
resolve spontaneously are not normally life-threatening. However,
prolonged seizures or seizures caused by another problem (for example, a head injury) are life-threatening and require urgent medical
intervention to control the seizure and treat the underlying problem.

Be aware that some people with epilepsy wear alert bracelets
or devices around their wrists, ankles, or necks to inform bystanders and medical staff that they have epilepsy. These may contain
emergency contact information, or instructions on what to do if
the person suffers from a seizure.

Medical Terminology

Epilepsy is a medical condition that causes recurrent seizures.

Signs and Symptoms of a Generalized Seizure

- Collapse and reduced level of consciousness
- Violent shaking episode (convulsion)
- Abnormal breathing
- Incontinence
- Tongue biting

First Aid Treatment for a Generalized Seizure

1. Remove any hazards from the area around the victim to make the scene safe.

2. Protect the victim's head.

3. Start timing the seizure.

4. Call EMS.

5. Once the jerking movements have stopped, open the victim's airway and place her in the recovery position (see The Recovery Position in Chapter 3).

6. Do not attempt to restrain the victim or place anything in her mouth (see sidebar, Common Seizure Myths).

7. Provide reassurance and monitor vital signs until emergency medical help arrives.

8. Take steps to protect the victim's dignity (for example, ensure bystanders move on), and the victim is kept warm and dry.

Some people with epilepsy will have occasional seizures and not require emergency medical help unless the seizure lasts for more than five minutes or they have multiple seizures. If you are unsure, always call EMS. Victims may be very tired following a seizure and want to sleep; this is normal as long as you're able to wake them up and they are not unconscious.

Common Seizure Myths

Unfortunately, there are many common myths circulating about the correct first aid treatment for a victim having a major epileptic seizure. Never place anything into the mouth of a victim having a seizure—this could cause blockage of her airway and result in serious harm. Never attempt to restrain a person having a seizure to stop the jerking movements. This is likely to cause harm to the victim or to you.

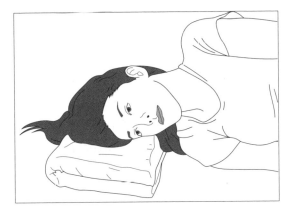

Protect a seizure victim's head to prevent a head injury.

Signs and Symptoms of a Focal Seizure

- Jerking movements in arms or legs
- Repetitive actions such as lip smacking or swallowing
- Hallucinations

First Aid Treatment for a Focal Seizure

1. Remove any hazards from the area around the victim to make the scene safe.

2. Start timing the seizure.

3. Provide reassurance until the seizure resolves.

4. Advise the victim to seek medical attention.

Be aware that some focal seizures may progress to major generalized seizures.

Diabetic Hyperglycemia (High Blood Sugar)

Diabetes is a common medical condition that causes elevated blood sugar levels in the body. Most of us know someone who is living with diabetes, as the condition is becoming much more common. There are two types of diabetes: type 1 and type 2. If left untreated, both types will cause dangerously high blood sugar levels (hyperglycemia). This can lead to life-threatening complications, including a diabetic coma. People living with diabetes are more at risk of heart attacks, strokes, and eye disease, especially if their blood sugar levels are persistently high. The main treatment for type 1 diabetes is the administration of insulin, via either regular injections or a continuous pump, and the regular monitoring of blood sugar levels. If a diabetic person misses a dose of insulin, then she becomes at risk of developing high blood sugar levels.

Medical Terminology

Hyperglycemia is the medical term for high blood sugar.

Signs and Symptoms of High Blood Sugar

- Excessive thirst
- Frequent urination
- Weight loss
- Visual disturbances
- Reduced level of consciousness

First Aid Treatment for High Blood Sugar

1. Call EMS.

2. If the victim becomes unconscious, open his airway and place him in the recovery position (see The Recovery Position in Chapter 3).

3. Encourage the victim to record his own blood sugar reading and act upon this if able to do so.

4. Provide reassurance and monitor vital signs until emergency medical help arrives.

5. Don't attempt to administer insulin unless you are specifically trained and authorized to do so.

Diabetic Hypoglycemia
(Low Blood Sugar)

Diabetes is a common medical condition that causes elevated blood sugar levels in the body. In the previous section, we looked at the symptoms and treatment of elevated blood sugar levels (hyperglycemia). In this section, we'll discuss what happens when blood sugar levels fall too low. Why might this happen? The main treatment for type 1 diabetes is the administration of insulin, via either regular injections or a continuous pump, and the regular monitoring of blood sugar levels. Type 2 diabetes may also be treated with insulin, often in combination with oral medications. People who administer insulin for diabetes (either type 1 or type 2) are at risk of developing low blood sugar levels. This can occur if too much insulin is administered or the person misses a meal after taking his or her insulin.

Medical Terminology

Hypoglycemia is the term for low blood sugar.

Testing Blood Sugar Levels

People with diabetes may carry a portable blood sugar monitoring kit. This allows them to check their blood sugar levels and can detect hyper- and hypoglycemia.

Signs and Symptoms of Low Blood Sugar

- Change in behavior (for example, irritability and aggression); these symptoms can mimic alcohol intoxication
- Confusion
- Excessive sweating
- Headache
- Reduced level of consciousness
- Seizures

First Aid Treatment for Low Blood Sugar

1. If the victim is conscious and able to swallow, give sugar by mouth using glucose tablets or a sugary drink.

2. Monitor the victim for ten to fifteen minutes; the symptoms should gradually resolve.

3. Encourage the victim to test his own blood sugar levels if he is able to do so.

4. If the symptoms do not resolve, or the victim deteriorates, call EMS.

Do not give sugar to a victim who is not fully conscious, or who is unable to swallow. There is a risk of the victim choking in this situation. Instead, immediately call EMS and be prepared to place the victim in the recovery position (see The Recovery Position in Chapter 3).

Poisoning

Poisoning occurs when a person comes into contact with a harmful substance. Our homes contain many potential poisons that can be dangerous if they are swallowed (ingested) or come into contact with our skin or eyes. In this section, we will look at four common poisoning situations and their first aid treatments. Always seek medical advice when dealing with a poisoning situation. In the United States, the National Poison Help Hotline (1-800-222-1222) provides free advice 24/7. If you are traveling abroad, other countries may have similar systems in place to provide advice regarding exposure to poisons.

Alcohol and Drugs

While many of us enjoy an alcoholic drink, excessive alcohol or recreational drug use can have a variety of harmful effects on the body. Acute alcohol or drug intoxication can be life-threatening. Unfortunately, every year more than two thousand Americans die from acute alcohol poisoning. Also, being intoxicated increases the risk of accidental death from other causes (for example, falling from a height or drowning), as alcohol interferes with our ability to make decisions and weigh risks. Alcohol intoxication can cause a victim to lose consciousness. This is a medical emergency like any other cause of unconsciousness. It is important not to brush off this situation as a victim being "just drunk." She may be at risk of blocking her airway. Also, be mindful that low blood sugar levels (see Diabetic Hypoglycemia earlier in this chapter) can mimic the symptoms of alcohol intoxication, so if the victim is diabetic, medical help should be sought to check his blood sugar levels.

Opioid poisoning is becoming an increasing problem across the United States. Opioids are strong painkilling medications available by prescription. In addition, heroin is a common illegal opioid that is highly addictive. The Centers for Disease Control and Prevention (CDC) estimates that in 2016 there were about 42,000 deaths due to opioid overdoses. An overdose of opioid medication causes a victim to become unconscious and stop breathing, quickly leading to death if treatment isn't administered. The main treatment of opioid overdose is administration of the drug naloxone (a common brand name is Narcan). Naloxone reverses the harmful effects of opioids and can be lifesaving in an emergency situation. There is increasing focus on training all emergency personnel in the use of naloxone, and in some communities, lay rescuers and opioid users are being trained in the use of this medicine. Naloxone can be administered using a nasal spray, meaning it can be used by rescuers with minimal training.

Signs and Symptoms of Alcohol or Drug Poisoning

- Vomiting
- Behavioral changes
- Confusion and aggression
- Reduced level of consciousness

First Aid Treatment for Alcohol or Drug Poisoning

1. Ensure the scene is safe for you to approach; victims who are intoxicated may be unpredictable or aggressive.

2. If the victim is unconscious, call EMS immediately; ensure her airway is open, and place her into the recovery position to reduce the risk of vomit blocking her airway (see The Recovery Position in Chapter 3).

3. If the victim is conscious, try to ask what she has taken and how much.

4. Seek medical assistance and ensure the victim is not left alone.

5. If an opioid overdose is suspected, administer nasal naloxone if available.

Household Cleaning Products

Household cleaning products contain strong chemicals and substances that can cause significant harm. Cleaning products may be accidentally swallowed (for example, by a child attracted by the bright colors of the product). Alternatively, cleaning products can splash onto the skin or into the eyes.

Signs and Symptoms of Household Cleaning Product Poisoning

- Vomiting
- Abdominal pain
- Burns
- Eye irritation
- Loss of vision
- Seizures
- Difficulty in breathing

First Aid Treatment for Household Cleaning Product Poisoning

1. Ensure the scene is safe for you to approach; do not expose yourself to the poison.

2. Try to determine what product the victim has come in contact with.

3. Call EMS if the victim appears unwell, has a seizure, is having trouble breathing, or is unconscious.

4. Otherwise, contact your local poison control center for advice (see sidebar, Contacting Poison Control).

5. If the poison has contaminated the eye, wash the eye with running water for at least fifteen to twenty minutes.

6. If the poison has contaminated the skin, remove any affected clothing and wash the area with running water for at least twenty minutes.

7. Ensure any runoff water from eye or skin washing is directed away from you and the victim.

Contacting Poison Control

In the United States you can contact the National Poison Help Hotline by calling 1-800-222-1222. The service is free and available twenty-four hours a day.

Don't Induce Vomiting

Do not induce vomiting unless specifically advised to do so by a medical professional or your local poison control center. Inducing vomiting may cause further damage to the victim's digestive tract when the poison is brought back up.

The Complete First Aid Pocket Guide

Carbon Monoxide

Carbon monoxide is a highly toxic gas generated by the incomplete burning of fuels such as coal, wood, and gas. Examples of situations that may generate carbon monoxide include campfires that haven't been put out properly and faulty boilers. The gas has no smell or taste, so it is very difficult to detect. Carbon monoxide poisoning is fatal, acts rapidly, and is responsible for about four hundred deaths a year in the United States.

Signs and Symptoms of Carbon Monoxide Poisoning

- Headache
- Dizziness
- Vomiting
- Confusion
- Reduced level of consciousness

First Aid Treatment for Carbon Monoxide Poisoning

1. Immediately call EMS and inform the 911 operator about the risk of carbon monoxide gas.

2. Do not enter a situation where you may put yourself at risk of carbon monoxide exposure.

3. If safe to do so, instruct the victim to move away from the potential source of carbon monoxide and into fresh air.

4. If the victim is unconscious and not breathing normally, update EMS and commence cardiopulmonary resuscitation (CPR) if safe to do so (see Cardiopulmonary Resuscitation (CPR) in Chapter 3).

5. Provide reassurance and monitor vital signs until emergency medical help arrives.

Protect Your Family with a Carbon Monoxide Alarm

Carbon monoxide gas is invisible and has no smell. This makes the gas deadly and difficult to detect. You can protect yourself by investing in a carbon monoxide alarm at home, especially if you have an open fire or generator.

Food Poisoning

Food poisoning occurs when we eat food contaminated with harmful bacteria. Many of us have experienced the unpleasant effects of food poisoning at some point in our lives. Common bacteria that cause food poisoning include norovirus, E. coli, and campylobacter. Incorrect storage or preparation of food (for example, undercooking meat or not refrigerating food) increases the risk of bacteria contaminating the food. Poor hand hygiene is another cause of contamination, as bacteria are easily transferred from our hands onto the food we touch. Unfortunately, there's no specific first aid treatment for food poisoning. Instead you should try to prevent dehydration and seek medical assistance if the symptoms are not subsiding. Knowing when to seek medical assistance is important; while most mild cases of food poisoning will not cause major problems, children and the elderly are at risk of developing complications from bad cases of food poisoning. Unfortunately, every year there are a number of deaths in the United States from severe food poisoning. Don't delay in seeking medical assistance if you are worried about a victim with food poisoning.

Signs and Symptoms of Food Poisoning

- Diarrhea
- Vomiting
- Abdominal pain
- Loss of appetite
- High temperature (fever)

First Aid Treatment for Food Poisoning

1. Encourage the victim to drink fluids to prevent dehydration; commercially available oral rehydration solutions (ORS), which include essential salts and sugar, can be used.

2. Ensure you and the victim perform adequate handwashing to reduce the risk of the infection spreading.

3. Seek medical help if you are concerned that the symptoms are not subsiding or the victim has other medical problems.

Young children and the elderly are most at risk from food poisoning. Severe cases of food poisoning can lead to dehydration and require hospital admission. Seek help early if you are concerned about a victim with food poisoning.

Emergency Childbirth

Childbirth is a naturally occurring process, and thousands of babies are born each day without serious complications. Normally, childbirth occurs at a planned location (for example, at a birthing center or hospital, or at home with a midwife). Emergency childbirth occurs when childbirth takes place in an unplanned location (for example, at home or in a car on the way to the hospital). This is not an uncommon occurrence, as the process of giving birth (labor) can be very quick. Let's take a look at labor in more detail.

Labor can be divided into three main stages:

- **Stage 1:** The cervix relaxes in order to prepare for the baby passing through.
- **Stage 2:** The baby is born through contractions and the mother pushing.
- **Stage 3:** The afterbirth (placenta) is delivered.

Thankfully, complications from childbirth are now rare. However, if a complication occurs it can be life-threatening for mother and baby. For example, severe blood loss after birth is a serious medical emergency that requires urgent assistance to stop the bleeding and prevent shock. Emergency 911 operators can provide specific instructions to recognize and manage complications of childbirth over the telephone. Always call EMS if concerned and follow the instructions of the operator carefully.

When dealing with an emergency childbirth situation, your main focus should be on remaining calm and supporting the mother. There are very few interventions you need to perform unless specifically advised to by an emergency 911 operator or a medical professional. Try to gather some clean towels to dry the baby with when he or she is born; these can also be used to keep the baby warm.

Signs and Symptoms of Childbirth

- The presence of regular strong contractions
- A sudden gush of fluid from the vagina (known as water breaking)
- Lower back pain

First Aid Treatment for Emergency Childbirth

1. Call EMS or a midwife.

2. Remain calm and reassuring.

3. Maintain the mother's dignity and control the scene (for example, ensure any bystanders move on).

4. Assist the mother into the most comfortable position, usually lying down.

5. Childbirth should occur naturally. Do not pull on the baby's head to speed up delivery. Encourage the mother to push with each contraction.

6. Receive the baby with a clean towel or sheet.

7. Thoroughly dry the baby and place him or her on the mother's chest. Ensure the newborn baby is kept warm.

8. Do not cut the umbilical cord.

If the baby does not appear to be breathing normally, attempt to stimulate the baby by drying and warming. Ensure the airway is open and clear. Check for the presence of normal breathing. If the baby is not breathing normally, immediately update EMS and begin cardiopulmonary resuscitation (see Pediatric Cardiopulmonary Resuscitation (CPR) in Chapter 8).

The afterbirth (placenta) will deliver naturally after the child is born. This process can take up to sixty minutes. Never pull on the umbilical cord to speed up delivery of the afterbirth.

Severe Blood Loss

Uncontrollable vaginal bleeding following childbirth is a medical emergency, and you should not delay in calling for EMS if the mother is bleeding. She may develop signs and symptoms of shock (see Shock in Chapter 6). While awaiting the arrival of EMS, uterine massage can be performed as a temporary measure:

1. Explain to the mother that you are going to place your hands on her abdomen.

2. Firmly massage the lower abdomen.

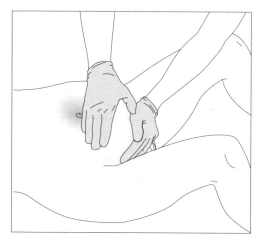

Perform a uterine massage to control severe blood loss after childbirth.

Chapter Eight
PEDIATRIC EMERGENCIES AND ILLNESSES

IN THIS CHAPTER, we're going to focus on common illnesses and emergency situations involving babies and children. Many first aid techniques, such as those used to treat minor injuries (see Chapter 4), are the same for children and adults. However, there are key differences in the lifesaving skills of CPR and managing choking, and you need to be aware of these differences. In addition, children can develop certain medical conditions (for example, croup) that are not seen in adults. If you look after children on a regular basis or you are a parent, you should sign up for an accredited pediatric first aid and CPR class in your area (see www.redcross.org/take-a-class or check with your local fire department), so you can have hands-on practice in these emergency first aid techniques. You never know when you might need to use them! Let's start off by looking at how to communicate with and assess the unwell child in a first aid situation.

Looking After an Unwell Child or Baby

Looking after an unwell child can be challenging, as every parent or guardian knows. Unwell or injured children are often frightened and irritable and may not cooperate with your instructions. Nonverbal children are difficult to assess, as they cannot describe the symptoms they are experiencing or the events prior to the incident. You should be aware that children can deteriorate rapidly from a serious illness, so it is always important to seek medical assistance if you are concerned about an unwell child.

Children are not simply small adults and they develop different medical problems than adults. For example, children are very unlikely to have a heart attack but they are very prone to developing problems with their breathing such as croup and bronchiolitis. In addition, you need to be aware that normal vital signs such as respiratory and pulse rates in a child and baby are much quicker than in an adult. We've listed the average normal ranges in the sidebar, Normal Pulse and Respiratory Rates, although these may vary slightly from child to child.

Communicating with an Unwell Child

It is important to gain the trust of a child who is unwell. She will understandably be frightened. Try these techniques to build trust and communicate with an unwell child.

- Drop down to the child's level; don't tower over her.
- Use easy-to-understand words and phrases (for example, a child may understand "hurt" but not "pain").
- Remain calm and in control of the situation; children will pick up if you display fear or anxiety.
- Provide lots of positive reinforcement and praise to the child.
- If you need to examine her or apply a bandage, try acting it out on Mom or Dad first to show the child what's involved.

Normal Pulse and Respiratory Rates

Children and babies will have different normal vital signs than adults (see Measuring Vital Signs in Chapter 1). These values are highly variable and will depend on the exact age of the child, her emotional state, and whether she is awake or asleep. As a rough guide, the average pulse and respiratory rates decrease as the child grows older and enters adulthood.

- Less than 1 year: Pulse 100–160; respiratory rate 30–40
- 1–2 years: Pulse 100–150; respiratory rate 25–35
- 2–5 years: Pulse 95–140; respiratory rate 20–25
- 5–12 years: Pulse 75–120; respiratory rate 18–25
- More than 12 years: As per adults

Recognizing an Unwell Child or Baby

A child or baby who is unwell may display some of the following features:

- Irritability or being inconsolable
- Reduced oral intake of fluid and food
- Reduced urine output; in babies, fewer wet diapers
- Quietness and withdrawal
- In babies, reduced muscle tone (floppy)
- Pale and mottled skin (patchy and irregular colors)
- Difficulty in breathing

You must not delay in seeking urgent medical help if you are concerned about an unwell child.

Assessing an Unresponsive Child or Baby

When assessing an unresponsive child or baby, use the DR ABC action plan in order to remember the correct first aid steps. We discussed the DR ABC plan for adults already (see Chapter 3); in this section, we will look at the modifications you need to make when assessing an unresponsive child or baby.

DR ABC Action Plan

- **D**anger
- **R**esponse
- **A**irway
- **B**reathing
- **C**PR (if required)

Danger

This remains the same as for an adult victim. Check for any hazards and ensure the scene is safe for you to approach before giving first aid. If the scene is too dangerous, stay back and call for EMS.

Response

To check for a response in a child, shout in both ears and tap him on the shoulders. In a baby, shout and flick the bottom of his foot in order to gain a response. Never shake a child or baby. If a baby or child is unconscious, immediately call EMS if you have not already done so.

Airway

In children, open the airway using the "head tilt chin lift" maneuver described in Chapter 3.

In babies, the procedure to open the airway is not the same as for adults and older children. The neck and throat of a baby are still developing, and the structures move differently than those of adults. The correct way to open the airway of a baby is to place the head in the neutral position as shown in the illustration. Do not tilt the baby's head backward, as this will obstruct the airway. In addition, take care not to apply any pressure to the neck of the baby; this can also block the airway.

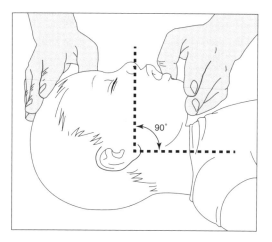

The correct position to open a baby's airway.

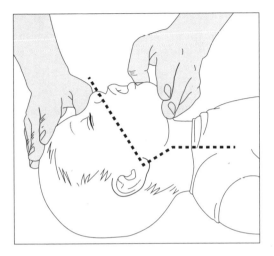

The incorrect position to open a baby's airway.

Breathing

As with adults, check for the presence of normal breathing for up to ten seconds. To do this, place your cheek just above the victim's mouth and look at his chest. Feel for exhaled air on the side of your cheek, look for the chest rising and falling, and listen for the sounds of breathing. The occasional gasp is not normal breathing.

CPR

As with adults, the last step of the DR ABC action plan is deciding whether you should begin CPR.

The Child or Baby Is Not Breathing

If the child or baby is not breathing normally, update EMS and immediately begin CPR. We'll cover how to perform CPR on babies and small children in the next section.

The Child or Baby Is Breathing

If the child or baby is breathing normally but is unconscious, perform a quick check to see if there is any major life-threatening bleeding. If you don't suspect a neck or back injury, the child should be rolled into the recovery position (see The Recovery Position in Chapter 3). Small babies can be cradled on their sides, with their heads slightly downward. This position keeps the airway open and protected until emergency medical help arrives.

Pediatric Cardiopulmonary Resuscitation (CPR)

This situation is every parent's worst nightmare: their baby or child has stopped breathing and needs urgent resuscitation. You need to act quickly to give emergency aid to the child and summon expert medical help. If a baby or child is not breathing normally, immediately begin cardiopulmonary resuscitation (CPR). The baby or child is likely to have suffered cardiac arrest, in which the heart has stopped pumping blood through the body. Ensure EMS has been updated so that the most appropriate emergency resources can be deployed to your location.

The key difference between adult CPR and pediatric CPR is the importance of rescue breathing. In adults, cardiac arrest is most likely caused by a problem with the heart (such as a heart attack). When adults suffer cardiac arrest, they still have a store of oxygen in their bloodstream. Therefore, the emphasis with adult victims is on performing high-quality, effective chest compressions in order to push this oxygenated blood through the body. Rescue breaths are less important and are only recommended for trained rescuers. Let's consider how children are different.

A child or baby is much less likely to suffer cardiac arrest from an underlying heart problem. Heart attacks in children are incredibly rare. The most common cause of pediatric cardiac arrest is a problem with breathing (for example, an acute asthma attack). Therefore, in a pediatric cardiac arrest situation, the victim is likely to be deprived of oxygen. As a result, rescue breathing is much more important during pediatric CPR.

The ratio of chest compressions to rescue breaths is the same as for an adult victim. Deliver two rescue breaths after each set of thirty chest compressions.

Don't forget the parents when dealing with this terrible situation. They are likely to be distraught and anxious. If possible, explain to them what you are doing and provide reassurance until EMS arrives to take over.

Child CPR (Ages 1 to Puberty)

When performing CPR on a child, chest compressions require less force than on an adult. It is acceptable to use one hand when delivering compressions. However, a large child may require the two-handed technique to achieve effective chest compression depth. Deliver chest compressions at the same rate as for an adult victim (100 to 120 chest compressions per minute) and in the same location (center of the chest). The depth of chest compressions on a child should be approximately one third the depth of the chest.

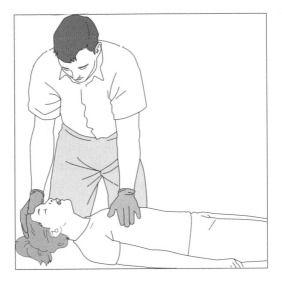

One-handed CPR can be used on a small child.

Rescue breaths for a child will require less force than for an adult victim. Ensure the child's airway is open and make a seal over her mouth. Use a disposable resuscitation face shield if available. Blow air in until the child's chest rises, then stop. Deliver two rescue breath attempts before immediately resuming chest compressions. If two rescuers are present, one can perform chest compressions and the other perform rescue breathing in order to minimize the interruption in chest compressions.

Baby CPR (Ages 0–1)

When performing CPR on a baby, chest compressions should be done by placing the pads of two fingers in the center of the baby's chest. Deliver chest compressions at the same rate as for an adult victim (100 to 120 chest compressions per minute). The depth of chest compressions on a baby should be approximately one third the depth of the chest.

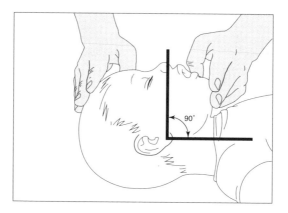

Open the baby's airway by lifting the baby's chin and holding the head in the neutral position.

When performing rescue breaths on a baby, you may need to make a seal over the baby's mouth and nose. Take care not to extend the neck when performing rescue breathing, as this will close off the airway. Breathe in only until the baby's chest rises; this will require just a small puff of air. Do not overinflate a baby's lungs.

Automated External Defibrillators (AEDs)

Standard AEDs can be used on children over eight years old. For children under eight, specialized pediatric defibrillator pads are recommended. However, an AED should not be used on children under one year old. See Chapter 3 for more information on how to use an automated external defibrillator on a victim in cardiac arrest.

Look After Yourself

Dealing with a pediatric CPR situation is a traumatic experience for all rescuers involved, especially lay rescuers and bystanders. Unless you work in a healthcare environment, you are unlikely to have performed CPR for real. You need to be aware of your own state of mind and mental health after an incident occurs. Remember, you are not invincible, and seeking help is not a sign of weakness!

Pediatric Choking

Kids love putting things they shouldn't in their mouths. It's their way of interacting with, exploring, and learning from the environment around them. Unfortunately, this makes them vulnerable to suffering from a choking episode. Food, too, can be a choking hazard for children; tragically, in the United States a child dies approximately every five days from choking on food. Children under the age of five are most at risk from accidental choking. All parents and caregivers should know how to manage a choking emergency. Prompt first aid measures can dislodge the object and unblock the airway. Let's start by looking at the signs and symptoms of choking.

Signs and Symptoms of Pediatric Choking

- Clutching the throat or chest
- Appearing distressed or panicked
- Difficulty in breathing
- Coughing
- Wheezing or grunting noises
- Turning pale or blue
- Reduced level of consciousness

If choking continues, the victim will become unconscious and stop breathing.

First Aid for a Choking Baby (Ages 0–1)

The emergency treatment for a choking baby is different because you cannot deliver abdominal thrusts to a baby. Instead, you should give back blows and chest compressions to attempt to dislodge the object:

1. Immediately call EMS.

2. Lay the baby down on your thigh with her head supported downward. Deliver five back blows to the baby, using the palm of your hand in the center of the baby's back. Check to see if the object has been dislodged after each blow.

3. Turn the baby over on your thigh while supporting her head.

4. Deliver up to five chest compressions. Place two fingers in the center of the chest and push inward and upward.

5. Repeat the cycle of back blows and chest compressions until the object is dislodged.

6. If the baby loses consciousness, assess whether she is breathing normally. If she is not breathing normally, immediately update EMS and commence cardiopulmonary resuscitation (CPR) until the arrival of medical help (see Pediatric Cardiopulmonary Resuscitation (CPR) earlier in this chapter).

Do not perform abdominal thrusts on a baby. Do not place your fingers blindly into the baby's mouth to attempt to remove the object as you could accidentally push the object farther down and worsen the choking situation. If you can easily see an object protruding from the mouth, you can attempt to carefully remove it. It can seem unnatural, but remember chest compressions and back blows need to be delivered with enough force to dislodge the object and save the baby's life.

First Aid for a Choking Child (Ages 1 to Puberty)

The emergency treatment for a child is the same as for an adult victim. The first step in helping a choking child is to establish whether there is complete or partial blockage of his airway. If the child can speak and cough then the blockage is only partial, as air is still able to move in and out of the lungs. If this is the case, then you should:

1. Encourage the child to cough to dislodge the object.

2. Provide reassurance and monitor the child.

3. Call EMS if the symptoms do not quickly resolve.

If the child is unable to speak or cough, then there is a complete obstruction of the airway. This is a life-threatening medical emergency requiring urgent first aid intervention. You should:

1. Immediately call EMS.

2. Deliver abdominal thrusts (Heimlich maneuver):

   a. Stand or kneel behind the child.

   b. Put your arms around his body, making a fist with one hand, and place this just above the victim's belly button.

   c. Grasp this fist with your other hand and firmly pull inward and upward.

3. Continue giving abdominal thrusts until emergency medical help arrives or the object is dislodged.

4. If the child loses consciousness, assess whether he is breathing normally. If he is not breathing normally, immediately update EMS and commence cardiopulmonary resuscitation (CPR) until the arrival of medical help (see Cardiopulmonary Resuscitation (CPR) in Chapter 3).

Any child who has suffered a serious choking episode should be assessed by a medical professional. Abdominal thrusts carry a risk of internal organ damage and bleeding, and therefore these victims need an urgent medical assessment.

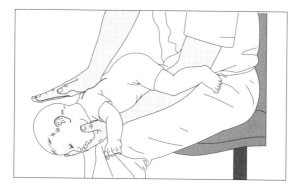

The correct position to deliver back blows to a choking baby.

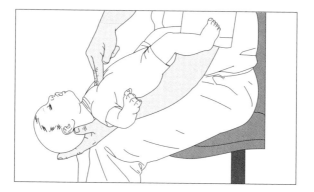

The correct position to deliver chest compressions to a choking baby.

Foreign Object Lodged in Ear

Children, especially toddlers, are at risk of putting small objects in their ears just like in their mouths. Anything small enough to fit in the ear can become lodged; common objects for this to happen with include pieces of food and small plastic toys. Insects lodged in the ear are another relatively common situation, and this can be incredibly distressing for the child. Often the symptoms of a foreign object are not noticed immediately, especially if the child cannot communicate his symptoms. Increasing pain or signs of an ear infection such as discharge may be the only signs of a foreign object lodged in the ear.

You may be able to carefully remove an easily visible object at home with tweezers; however, deeper objects will require medical assessment and removal. You should only attempt to remove an object that is easily visible and accessible. Never use instruments to try to examine the ear at home, as you risk pushing the object farther in and causing more pain and damage. If in doubt, seek medical attention before attempting to remove an embedded object, especially if you suspect the object has been in the ear for a long time.

Small button batteries are becoming an increasingly common foreign object found in children's ears due to their widespread use in household items. These batteries can cause significant burns and leak strong chemicals, resulting in permanent skin damage. Unfortunately, many button batteries are small enough to fit into a child's ear. If you suspect a button battery is in a child's ear, you should seek urgent medical attention to enable a quick removal of the battery.

Signs and Symptoms of a Foreign Object in the Ear

- Ear pain
- Hearing loss
- Discharge from the ear
- Repeated pulling or tugging at the ear

First Aid Treatment for a Foreign Object in the Ear

1. If the object is easily visible and hanging out, attempt to grasp it with tweezers to remove it.

2. Never use cotton swabs or other instruments in the ear. This risks pushing the object farther in. Only attempt to remove the object if it can be easily seen and grasped with tweezers.

3. Lay the child with the affected side down to try to dislodge the object.

4. If an insect is in the ear, use baby or olive oil to drown it (see sidebar, Dealing with Insects) and don't use tweezers, as this could cause the insect to crawl deeper into the ear.

5. Seek medical attention if you are unable to remove the object, there is discharge from the ear, or the child experiences hearing loss.

6. Seek urgent medical attention if the object is a battery. These require quick removal to prevent burns and tissue damage.

Remember, one of the aims in first aid is to prevent worsening of the victim's condition (see Chapter 1). If unsure, always seek specialist help for removal of a foreign object rather than risk making the situation worse.

Dealing with Insects

A live insect in the ear is incredibly uncomfortable and will be distressing for the child. Warm (not hot) baby or olive oil can be used to drown the insect and attempt to float it out. Turn the child's head to the side with the affected ear upward. Carefully pour about a tablespoon of oil into the ear to kill the insect. The ear can then be placed downward to allow the oil, and hopefully the insect, to float out. Do not use oil to attempt to remove objects other than insects, and never perform this if there is discharge from the ear, as this may indicate that the eardrum has been perforated.

Foreign Object Lodged in Nose

Our noses are complex structures with multiple folds of tissue and bone, and as a result it is easy for an object to become lodged deep in the nose and require removal by a medical professional. Remember, the nose is connected to the throat and the airway; therefore there is always a risk of choking with foreign objects in the nose, especially if they are accidentally pushed farther in. Like foreign objects in the ear, the object may be there for some time before the child starts to show any symptoms such as bleeding or persistent discharge.

Small button batteries are becoming an increasingly common foreign object found in children's noses due to their widespread use in household items. These batteries can cause significant burns and leak strong chemicals, resulting in permanent skin damage. Unfortunately, many button batteries are small enough to fit into a child's nose. If you suspect a button battery is in a child's nose, you should seek urgent medical attention to enable a quick removal of the battery.

Signs and Symptoms of a Foreign Object in the Nose

- Nose pain
- Recurrent nosebleeds
- Discharge from the nose
- Persistent congested or blocked nose

First Aid Treatment for a Foreign Object in the Nose

1. If the object is easily visible and hanging out, attempt to grasp it with tweezers to remove it.

2. If the object is not visible, do not put cotton swabs or other instruments into the nose, as you risk pushing the foreign body farther in.

3. Pinch the unaffected nostril and ask the child to lean forward and blow her nose; this may dislodge the object.

4. Seek medical advice if the object is not visible, you are unable to remove the object, or there is persistent discharge from the nose.

5. Seek urgent medical attention if the object is a battery. These require quick removal to prevent burns and tissue damage.

Remember, one of the aims in first aid is to prevent worsening of the victim's condition (see Chapter 1). If unsure, always seek specialist help for removal of the foreign object rather than risk making the situation worse.

Croup

Croup is a common condition that causes inflammation of the windpipe in babies and young children. This inflammation causes problems with the child's breathing and a characteristic barking cough. Croup is most common in children ages three months to six years, but it can occur in older children too. The most common cause of croup is a viral infection. Mild croup often improves with steroid treatment prescribed by a medical professional; however, severe cases may require hospital admission and treatment to support the child's breathing. Always seek medical advice if you are concerned about a child's breathing.

Medical Terminology

The medical term for croup is *laryngotracheobronchitis*.

Signs and Symptoms of Croup

- Barking cough, often described as "seal like"
- Hoarse voice
- Difficulty in breathing
- Symptoms of a cold: runny nose, sore throat, high temperature (fever)

The symptoms of croup tend to be worse during the night or when the child becomes upset.

First Aid Treatment for Croup

1. Provide reassurance to the child and keep her calm to reduce the work of breathing.

2. Position her so that she is sitting upright.

3. Give regular fluids to avoid dehydration.

4. Seek medical advice; the child may require steroid treatment to reduce the inflammation in the windpipe.

5. Call EMS if the child appears distressed or turns blue or floppy or if you are concerned her breathing is deteriorating.

What About Steam?

In the past, parents were advised to place their child in a steam-filled environment to relieve the symptoms of croup. This is no longer advised as research has shown that steam does not improve symptoms of croup. In addition, there have been reported cases of children being badly burned from prolonged steam exposure by parents trying to treat croup.

Bronchiolitis

Bronchiolitis is a common viral infection that causes inflammation and swelling of the small airways (bronchioles) in children's lungs. This is different from croup, which affects the larger wind-pipe. The swelling in the small airways causes the child to work harder to move air in and out of his lungs. Despite being very common, this condition is not as well known as other childhood illnesses; you might not have heard of it. Bronchiolitis is most common in young children under the age of two and is one of the most common reasons in this age group for hospital admission. Bronchiolitis is most commonly seen in the winter months and peaks between December and March. Most mild cases of bronchiolitis will settle with no medical treatment; however, this disease can be serious and cause major problems with breathing in young children. Life-threatening cases of bronchiolitis may require the child to be admitted to a pediatric intensive care unit (PICU) to support his breathing. As a result, you should never delay seeking medical help if you are concerned about a child's breathing. Bronchiolitis is more likely to cause complications if a child was born early (premature) or has a preexisting heart condition. These children often need to be admitted to the hospital for close monitoring by a pediatrician.

Medical Terminology

The most common cause of bronchiolitis is a virus called *respiratory syncytial virus (RSV)*.

Signs and Symptoms of Bronchiolitis

- Runny or congested nose
- High temperature (fever)
- Persistent cough
- A wheezing sound
- Difficulty in breathing
- Reduced appetite

First Aid Treatment for Bronchiolitis

1. Give regular fluids to avoid dehydration.

2. Simple antifever medication (for example, acetaminophen) can be used to reduce high temperatures (fever).

3. Seek medical advice.

4. Call EMS if the child appears distressed or turns blue or floppy or if you are concerned his breathing is deteriorating.

Chicken Pox

Chicken pox is a common, but unpleasant, viral infection that affects many children at some point in childhood. Fortunately, due to vaccination not all children will be affected. The virus causes a characteristic red rash, followed by small blisters all over the body. Most cases of chicken pox are mild, and the child will make a good recovery within a week or so. However, in rare cases, chicken pox can cause serious lung infections (pneumonia) or affect the brain and spinal cord. A relatively common complication is infection of the blisters by bacteria, causing a wound infection. If this occurs, antibiotic treatment may be required to control the infection.

Luckily, the majority of healthy children with mild chicken pox will recover with no treatment. However, very young children or children with other medical problems are more at risk of developing complications and may require treatment with antiviral medication. Chicken pox is very contagious and is easily spread between people. Chicken pox becomes contagious around one to two days before the rash and small blisters appear. A child with chicken pox is at risk of transmitting the disease until all the small blisters have dried up and crusted over.

Medical Terminology

The virus that causes chicken pox is the *varicella zoster virus (VZV)*. This virus is also responsible for causing shingles in adults. The risk of shingles can be avoided if children are vaccinated early and never get chicken pox.

Signs and Symptoms of Chicken Pox

- Red rash with small fluid-filled blisters
- High temperature (fever)
- Lethargy

First Aid Treatment for Chicken Pox

1. Encourage regular baths and use calamine lotion to reduce the itching from the blisters.

2. Discourage scratching, and trim the child's nails to reduce the chances of skin damage and infection of the blisters.

3. Simple painkillers such as acetaminophen can be used to control pain and fever. Don't give aspirin to children.

4. Monitor for dehydration and encourage fluid intake.

5. Avoid contact with other children, pregnant women, and people with weakened immune systems until all the blisters have dried and crusted.

6. Seek medical advice if you are concerned or there are any worrying features (see sidebar, When to Seek Medical Help).

When to Seek Medical Help

In healthy children, mild cases of chicken pox often do not require treatment. However, chicken pox has the potential to cause serious complications, especially in very young children, children with chronic diseases, or those with weakened immune systems. You should seek medical help if:

- The child is a newborn.
- There is evidence of dehydration (see Dehydration later in this chapter).
- The blisters become red, painful, or pus filled. This may be a sign of infection requiring antibiotics.
- The child has difficulty breathing or develops a severe cough.
- The child has a severe headache, sensitivity to light, or neck stiffness.
- The child displays any other symptoms that cause you to be concerned.

Febrile Seizures

A febrile seizure is a seizure caused by an elevated body temperature (fever) in a child. Febrile seizures commonly occur in children ages three months to six years old. Between 2 and 4 percent of children will experience at least one febrile seizure by the age of five. Febrile seizures are very frightening for parents to watch but rarely cause any permanent harm or disability to a child, and most last less than five minutes. All children who have had their first seizure should be assessed by a medical professional in order to rule out other potential causes of seizures. Most febrile seizures will stop without medical treatment; however, in some cases medication may be required to stop the seizures.

Medical Terminology

Febrile convulsion is another term used to refer to a febrile seizure.

Signs and Symptoms of a Febrile Seizure

- Loss of consciousness
- Stiffening of muscles
- Repetitive jerking movements of the arms and legs
- Incontinence
- High temperature (fever)

First Aid Treatment for a Febrile Seizure

1. Protect the child from injury by placing pillows or other padding around her.

2. Remove excessive clothing and open a window to cool the child.

3. Once the seizure is over, place the child on her side and ensure her airway is open.

4. Do not attempt to restrain the child or place anything in her mouth.

5. Seek medical assistance, or call EMS if the seizure is prolonged, the child has multiple seizures, or it is her first seizure.

Dehydration

When a baby or child is unwell, he is at risk of developing dehydration, as he has less fluid reserves than adults. Dehydration occurs when the body loses more fluid than is replaced. A baby or child may lose excessive fluid through having a high temperature (fever) or diarrhea and vomiting. Severe dehydration is life-threatening for babies and young children, as it affects the balance of salts and minerals in the bloodstream and can lead to complications such as kidney failure. Always be vigilant and seek medical advice if you are concerned a baby or child is becoming dehydrated. In severe cases, he will need to be admitted to the hospital for blood tests and fluid replacement through a drip.

Signs and Symptoms of Dehydration

- Lack of energy
- Irritability
- Dry lips and mouth
- Decreased urine output (in babies, fewer wet diapers)
- Dark-colored urine
- Cool skin
- Sunken eyes
- Skin tenting (see sidebar, Spotting Dehydration Using Skin)

Spotting Dehydration Using Skin

You can test for dehydration in a child by looking for skin tenting. Children's skin is normally elastic and stretchy. However, dehydration can cause the skin to become less elastic as the underlying tissues become dehydrated. This can be tested for by pinching a fold of skin, typically on the back of the hand, and then releasing the skin. If the skin remains elevated and only slowly flattens this is known as skin tenting. The presence of skin tenting indicates moderate to severe dehydration in a child.

First Aid Treatment for Dehydration

1. Encourage the child or baby to drink small amounts often.

2. Use a commercially available oral rehydration solution (ORS) to replace lost salt and sugar.

3. Seek urgent medical advice if the child or baby does not improve or continues to lose excessive fluid.

Chapter Nine
ENVIRONMENTAL CONDITIONS

IF YOU ENJOY OUTDOOR ACTIVITIES such as hiking, climbing, or water sports, you should be aware of the warning signs of common environmental conditions such as heatstroke and hypothermia. Our bodies are designed to work effectively at a specific temperature of around 98.6°F (37°C). Being exposed to extreme weather can disrupt this ideal temperature and lead to overheating or hypothermia. Both of these conditions can be life-threatening if steps are not taken quickly to correct the temperature disturbance. In addition, you should be prepared to deal with other outdoor emergency situations such as lightning strikes, which are more common than you might think. In this chapter, we'll show you how to recognize and treat common conditions that you might encounter when exposed to the elements.

Hypothermia

Hypothermia occurs when a person's core body temperature drops to a dangerously low level. The signs and symptoms of hypothermia develop once the body temperature drops below 95°F (35°C). A temperature below 90°F (32°C) is classed as moderate hypothermia, and a temperature below 82°F (28°C) is severe hypothermia, which is life-threatening if the victim does not receive emergency care. Young children and the elderly are most at risk for developing hypothermia. Other risk factors include being intoxicated and certain prescription medications. While hypothermia is commonly associated with being outside in colder weather, this condition can also develop when a victim is in a home with inadequate heating. Correct first aid treatment of hypothermia is important in order to raise the body temperature and prevent the victim from slipping into a coma. Unfortunately, there are a number of common myths regarding the correct way to treat a hypothermic victim; we've highlighted them in the Common Hypothermia Myths sidebar.

Signs and Symptoms of Hypothermia

Mild to Moderate Hypothermia
- Shivering
- Lack of coordination and fine movements
- Confusion

Severe to Life-Threatening Hypothermia

- Shivering stops
- Reduced level of consciousness
- Rigid muscles

First Aid Treatment for Hypothermia

1. If the victim is outside or exposed to the elements, move her to a warm, dry place if possible. If this is not possible, seek shelter.

2. Call EMS and Search and Rescue if in a remote outdoor location.

3. Remove and replace any wet clothing.

4. If the victim is conscious and able to swallow safely, give her warm drinks with sugar and high-energy food (for example, a chocolate bar, a cereal bar, or an energy bar).

5. Cover the victim in warm layers (for example, blankets) and ensure her head is covered. If possible, cover the face loosely to prevent frostbite from developing on her ears or cheeks but take care not to restrict the victim's breathing.

6. If available, place warm hot-water bottles or reusable heat packs in the victim's armpits and groin.

7. If the victim becomes unconscious, she will need to be placed in the recovery position to protect the airway (see The Recovery Position in Chapter 3).

8. Severe hypothermia can cause the heart to stop beating effectively. Be prepared to perform cardiopulmonary resuscitation (CPR) if the victim stops breathing normally (see Cardiopulmonary Resuscitation (CPR) in Chapter 3).

Be aware of your own safety. If in an outdoor situation, take appropriate steps to ensure you do not develop hypothermia and become a second victim.

Common Hypothermia Myths

There are a number of first aid myths regarding the correct treatment of hypothermia:

- Do not rub alcohol on the victim's skin. Doing this will not warm her up; instead it will draw blood away from the body's core and accelerate heat loss.
- Do not place the victim in a hot bath, as this will also draw blood away from the body's core. In addition, there is a risk of the victim sustaining a burn injury if she is placed in a tub of scalding hot water.
- Do not give the victim any drinks containing alcohol. Doing this will cause the blood vessels to dilate, and the body will lose more heat.

Frostbite

Anyone who works in cold environments or spends time outdoors in the cold needs to be aware of the risk of frostbite. Frostbite is caused by freezing of the skin and underlying tissue. The majority of cases of frostbite are preventable by wearing enough suitable warm clothing for the conditions. Toes, fingers, and the face are most at risk of developing frostbite, as these areas are farthest away from the body's core and therefore most at risk of freezing.

Frostbite is split into two main categories: superficial and deep. Superficial frostbite occurs when only the top layer of skin is frozen. This may cause blistering of the skin. Deep frostbite occurs when the underlying tissue is frozen. Deep frostbite can cause permanent damage to the skin and underlying muscle due to these structures freezing. There is a risk of infection, and the victim may require surgery to remove damaged tissue or, in severe cases, to amputate the affected limb.

Signs and Symptoms of Superficial Frostbite

- Numbness in the affected area
- Swelling
- Blistering of the skin

The early stages of frostbite can be easily missed because the initial symptom is numbness and loss of sensation in the affected area.

Signs and Symptoms of Deep Frostbite

- Blue colored skin
- Hard black skin
- Formation of an ulcer

First Aid Treatment for Frostbite

1. Seek medical assistance; rewarming a frostbite injury is very painful, and the victim may require strong painkillers and a thorough assessment of the frostbite injury.

2. Monitor the victim for the development of hypothermia (see Hypothermia earlier in this chapter) and move her to a warm, dry, sheltered place.

3. Remove any constricting items near the affected area, such as watches and rings, before the frostbitten area starts to swell.

If prompt medical assistance is not available:

1. Only consider rewarming if there is no risk of the affected area being refrozen.

2. To rewarm, place the affected area in warm water at 99–103°F (37–39°C); the rewarming process can take up to an hour and is complete when the affected area has returned to a normal color and sensation is restored.

3. Protect the area by applying a sterile dressing and cover to prevent refreezing.

The rewarming process is very painful for a victim. If possible, seek medical assistance to ensure adequate pain relief can be given to keep the victim comfortable.

Heatstroke

In contrast to hypothermia (low body temperature; see earlier section in this chapter), heatstroke is a life-threatening situation that occurs when the body becomes too hot and is unable to regulate temperature effectively. Heatstroke can be deadly, as the high body temperature causes vital organs to rapidly shut down. In addition, victims of heatstroke are often dehydrated because excessive fluid is lost through sweating. A victim of heatstroke has a high risk of dying unless immediate steps are taken to reduce his body temperature and restore lost fluid. Active cooling (for example, by using running water) is the main treatment in a heatstroke situation. All victims with suspected heatstroke need a thorough medical assessment, as they can develop complications affecting the heart, kidneys, and other vital organs. Children and the elderly are most at risk of developing heatstroke, so you need to be vigilant, especially during periods of hot weather. Heatstroke can also be brought on by exercising in very hot conditions, and athletes or outdoor workers should be aware of the risk of heatstroke and know how to spot the warning signs in their peers.

Signs and Symptoms of Heatstroke

- Hot and dry skin
- Body temperature above 105°F (41°C)
- Reduced level of consciousness and confusion
- Increased pulse and respiratory rate
- Extreme thirst

First Aid Treatment for Heatstroke

1. Immediately call EMS.
2. Move the victim to a cool and sheltered place.
3. Remove any excessive outer clothing.
4. Cool the victim by using cool (but not freezing) running water and by placing ice-packs in his groin and armpits.

The Complete First Aid Pocket Guide

5. If the victim is fully conscious and able to swallow, give him sips of cool water to drink.

6. If the victim becomes unconscious, he will need to be turned into the recovery position to protect the airway (see The Recovery Position in Chapter 3).

7. Be prepared to perform cardiopulmonary resuscitation (CPR) if the victim loses consciousness and stops breathing normally (see Cardiopulmonary Resuscitation (CPR) in Chapter 3).

Take care not to overcool the victim and cause hypothermia.

Sunburn

As something we've all experienced at some point in our lives, sunburn is very common. But how many of us actually perform simple first aid measures to help our skin recover properly from the burn? Sunburn is caused by exposure to ultraviolet (UV) radiation from the sun, which damages the superficial skin tissue. Sunburn is painful but often heals with no significant complications. However, prolonged exposure to UV radiation increases the risk of skin cancer and accelerates the aging process in the skin. Severe sunburn can occasionally cause significant burns that require specialist medical intervention. Prevention is always better than cure when considering sunburn; protect yourself and your family by taking appropriate steps to reduce sun exposure (see sidebar,

Protecting Yourself from Sunburn). Most sunburn can be treated at home with self-care measures. However, severe cases will require a medical assessment, especially if there are large blisters.

Protecting Yourself from Sunburn

- Apply sunscreen with a high SPF (sun protection factor) liberally over all areas of exposed skin.
- Reapply sunscreen after two hours or after any immersion in water.
- Wear appropriate clothing and cover exposed areas.
- Avoid being in the sun during the hottest part of the day (11 a.m.–3 p.m.).

Signs and Symptoms of Sunburn

- A history of exposure to direct sunlight
- Red, painful skin
- Peeling or blistering of the skin
- Itching

First Aid Treatment for Sunburn

1. Avoid further exposure to the sun.

2. Cool the skin with running water.

3. Apply after-sun lotion.

4. Encourage sips of water to prevent dehydration.

5. Do not burst any blisters that form. If a blister bursts on its own, gently clean the area to prevent infection and apply a sterile dressing. If the wound left by the burst blister is showing signs of infection, seek medical attention as soon as possible.

Burn Injury Myths

Like other types of burns, sunburns should be cooled only with running water to remove heat from the burn. There are many myths regarding the correct treatment of burns:

■ Do not apply toothpaste or butter to a burn. This will not cool the burn adequately and can introduce infection. The best method to cool a minor burn is with running water.

■ Do not burst blisters as this will increase the risk of infection in the burn.

■ Do not place ice on a minor burn to speed up the cooling process. This could cause freeze burns to the skin.

Lightning Strike

Being struck by lightning is not as rare as you might think. Around thirty people in the United States are killed each year by being hit by lightning. Many more victims are struck by lightning and survive. Statistics show only around 10 percent of lightning strikes are fatal. Lightning strikes can cause severe electrical burns and disrupt the electrical activity of the heart, causing cardiac arrest. The victim may be thrown to the ground and sustain further injuries, including head injuries or limb fractures.

If you find yourself caught outside in a thunderstorm, seek shelter immediately in a building or vehicle and stay there for at least thirty minutes after the storm has passed. If you can't find shelter quickly, avoid high ground and stay away from tall objects and water. Many people believe that crouching down is an effective way to stay safe during a thunderstorm; however, you are still at risk if you remain outdoors. Seeking shelter is the only effective way to protect yourself from a lightning strike. If no other shelter is available, a car will provide some limited protection from a lightning strike, although this isn't due to the rubber in the tires as most people believe. The metal body of a car will conduct the electricity from a lightning strike to the ground. Obviously, this only works when the car has a metal shell—unfortunately, a soft-top convertible will not keep you safe during a thunderstorm.

First Aid Treatment for a Lightning Strike

1. Consider your own safety, and take immediate shelter indoors if there is a risk of further lightning strikes.

2. Immediately call EMS.

3. The victim is safe to touch after a lightning strike; the body will not retain any electrical charge.

4. If the victim is conscious, assess for any injuries and burns. Monitor vital signs and provide reassurance until medical help arrives. Move the victim to shelter if safe to do so.

5. If the victim is unconscious, assess for the presence of normal breathing and commence cardiopulmonary resuscitation (CPR) if required (see Cardiopulmonary Resuscitation (CPR) in Chapter 3).

Drowning

Witnessing a drowning incident is terrifying. If a victim is successfully rescued from the water, there is inevitably much relief among bystanders and rescuers. However, most people don't realize that the victim is still at risk of serious medical complications. This is where you can help save her life. She may be out of the water, but she's not out of danger.

A victim may appear to have recovered from being in the water then suddenly deteriorate and become unwell. Why does this occur? First, the victim may develop hypothermia (dangerously low body temperature), especially if the water is very cold. Wet clothing causes a significant amount of heat loss and puts the victim at risk of hypothermia. If water has entered the victim's throat, there is a risk of the voice box going into spasm. This is a serious situation, since the spasm causes the victim's airway to close up and air can't enter the lungs. Advanced medical help is urgently required to protect the airway and stop the victim from suffocating.

If water has entered the victim's lungs, the water can irritate the lungs and cause breathing problems. Even a small volume of water entering the lungs can cause serious damage and impair breathing.

Always seek medical attention if a victim has been rescued from a drowning situation. If a victim has sustained lung damage, there's not much you can do in first aid to fix this. These victims need urgent specialist medical help to protect their airway and stop further lung damage.

Signs and Symptoms of Non-Fatal Drowning

- Difficulty in breathing
- Increased respiratory rate
- Coughing
- Chest pain
- Vomiting
- Pale, cold skin

First Aid Treatment for Non-Fatal Drowning

1. Immediately call EMS.

2. Provide reassurance and monitor vital signs until emergency medical help arrives.

3. Remove any wet clothing and monitor the victim closely for the development of hypothermia (see Hypothermia earlier in this chapter).

4. If the victim loses consciousness, assess whether she is breathing normally. If she is not breathing normally, immediately update EMS and commence cardiopulmonary resuscitation (CPR) until the arrival of medical help (see Cardiopulmonary Resuscitation (CPR) in Chapter 3).

Poison Ivy, Oak, and Sumac

If you're an avid gardener or backcountry hiker you are aware of the risks of coming into contact with poison ivy, oak, and sumac. Why do we need to watch out for these plants? Poison ivy, oak, and sumac all secrete a sticky oil called urushiol. This oil can cause an allergic reaction when it comes into contact with our skin. Some people are very sensitive to urushiol and can suffer significant skin reactions when they come into contact with poison ivy, oak, or sumac. The urushiol oil from these poisonous plants can also contaminate clothing and pets, leading to recurrent exposure and skin reactions. While uncomfortable, the skin reaction from poison ivy, oak, and sumac will often resolve with no treatment, although severe cases may require medical assessment. In rare cases, the victim may have a life-threatening allergy to urushiol oil, which causes anaphylaxis (see Anaphylaxis in Chapter 7). You also need to be aware of the significant risk of smoke from burning these plants. Burning poison ivy, oak, or sumac can cause toxic smoke, which if inhaled can lead to serious breathing problems and internal reactions. You should always seek urgent medical advice if a victim has been exposed to this toxic smoke, even if he appears to have no symptoms, as the toxic effects can be delayed.

Signs and Symptoms of Poison Ivy, Oak, and Sumac

- Red itchy rash
- Small fluid-filled blisters (in severe cases)

The rash is often delayed and may occur several hours after exposure; it can take around ten to fourteen days to fully heal. Watch out for signs and symptoms of a severe allergic reaction; these include:

- Difficulty in breathing
- Tongue swelling
- Facial swelling
- Reduced level of consciousness

First Aid Treatment for Poison Ivy, Oak, and Sumac

1. Call EMS if the victim has any difficulty in breathing, facial swelling, or a history of anaphylaxis.

2. Thoroughly scrub the affected skin with running water and soap to remove the oil causing the reaction.

3. Apply calamine lotion if the skin is itchy.

4. Oral antihistamines can reduce itching but may cause side effects such as drowsiness.

5. Don't burst any blisters that form, as this will increase the risk of infection.

6. Seek medical advice if the reaction is severe; steroids can be used in the treatment of severe cases of poison ivy, oak, and sumac.

7. Monitor the area for the signs and symptoms of infection (see sidebar, Watch Out for Infection).

Watch Out for Infection

Rashes and blisters from poison ivy, oak, and sumac are at risk of becoming infected, especially if the victim has been scratching the area. Watch out for these warning signs that may indicate an infected rash:

- Increasing pain
- A rapidly spreading red area around the rash
- Swelling
- Pus discharging from the small blisters
- High temperature (fever)
- Swollen glands near the rash

Do not delay seeking medical attention if you are concerned a rash is infected. If left untreated, the infection could spread to the bloodstream and cause blood poisoning (septicemia).

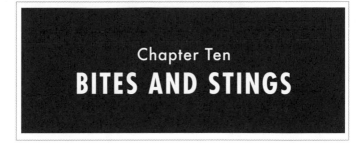

Chapter Ten
BITES AND STINGS

ANIMAL BITES AND INSECT STINGS are common scenarios you might encounter, especially if you are involved in outdoor activities and hobbies. Luckily, the majority of insect stings only cause us minor irritation and pain. However, in rare cases, the venom from an insect sting can cause a life-threatening major allergic reaction known as anaphylaxis. You should always monitor any victim of an insect sting for the signs and symptoms of anaphylaxis developing (see Chapter 7 for more information on how to recognize and treat anaphylaxis). People with a known severe allergy to insect stings should carry an epinephrine auto-injector (EpiPen) with them to use in the event of a severe reaction. If you hike in the backcountry, you should look out for tick bites as well as insect stings. Ticks can spread various diseases, including Lyme disease, and they should be removed as soon as possible to reduce the risk of infection.

Animal bites are becoming increasingly common, and the majority of these occur from domesticated animals such as dogs and cats. If dealing with an animal bite, you need to be aware of the risk of infection developing in the wound. Animals (and humans!) carry lots of germs in their mouths, which can cause serious wound infections. These wounds require thorough cleaning and an assessment by a medical professional. Basic first aid steps should focus on stopping the bleeding and cleaning the wound. Let's start this chapter by looking at animal bites in more detail and the correct first aid measures for the victim.

Animal Bites

Cats and dogs are responsible for the majority of animal bites. Dogs are not always man's best friend, and it is estimated more than four million Americans are bitten by a dog each year. Animal bites can cause deep puncture wounds to the skin and can easily become infected due to the germs that live in the animal's mouth. Serious dog bites can be life-threatening, especially for young children and babies. There is a risk of rabies from animal bites in developing countries, especially with bites from wild animals (see sidebar, What About Rabies?). Thankfully, rabies is now rare in North America. There are only a handful of cases in humans each year, and modern medical treatments are very effective in suspected cases.

Consider your own safety when dealing with an animal bite; you do not want to become a second victim! A frightened or distressed animal can be dangerous and unpredictable. Specialist help may be required to safely contain the animal and prevent further injuries.

The victim of an animal bite may have deep puncture wounds, so your first priority is to stem any major bleeding from the wound by applying firm, direct pressure. After this, the bite needs to be thoroughly cleaned if the bleeding has stopped and medical help sought. All animal bites should be assessed by a medical professional for consideration of antibiotic treatment and an assessment of the victim's immunization status. A tetanus shot may be recommended if the victim's tetanus immunizations are not up to date.

First Aid Treatment for an Animal Bite

1. Consider your own safety; do not attempt to deal with a dangerous animal unless you are trained and confident in managing animals.

2. If the wound is bleeding, apply direct pressure over the wound to stem the bleeding.

3. If the wound is not bleeding profusely, wash with running water and soap if available then apply antibiotic ointment and a sterile bandage.

4. Seek medical assistance.

5. Call EMS immediately if you are unable to control the bleeding, the victim is a child or baby, or the victim develops signs and symptoms of shock (see Shock in Chapter 6).

A serious dog attack, especially when the victim is a young child or baby, can be life-threatening. Do not delay in calling for EMS in this situation. If the dog is still loose, inform the 911 operator, as law enforcement may be required in order to contain the dog safely.

What About Rabies?

Rabies is a virus carried by infected animals in their saliva. The animal can transmit the virus to humans through a bite or scratch. The rabies virus causes inflammation of the brain and spinal cord resulting in serious symptoms and death if left untreated. Rabies may be found in wild animals but is now rare in domesticated animals in North America. The treatment for rabies involves the prompt administration of the rabies vaccine as soon as possible following suspected exposure to the virus.

Bites from Humans

Bites from a fellow human should be treated in the same way as a bite from a dog or a cat. The wound should be thoroughly cleaned, and medical advice sought. Human bites are also at a high risk of becoming infected due to the germs that live in our mouths and on our teeth.

Snakebites

Although many people have a fear of snakes, the chances of being bitten by a snake in the United States are very low. Luckily, fatalities from snakebites are rare, with only a handful reported each year. Snakes do not always inject venom when they bite, and when this occurs, it is called a dry bite. Although painful, dry bites do not come with the risks of the snake venom entering the body. Snake venom can cause a range of symptoms depending on the type of snake and the amount of venom that has entered the body (see sidebar, Signs and Symptoms of Snake Venom Toxicity). Identifying the snake involved can be very useful to help doctors guide the treatment given to the victim of a bite; however, do not risk being bitten by attempting to capture or kill the snake.

Signs and Symptoms of Snake Venom Toxicity

- Extreme pain and swelling around the bite
- Numbness around the affected area
- Muscle weakness
- Blurred vision
- Excessive drooling
- Vomiting
- Decreased level of consciousness

First Aid Treatment for a Snakebite

1. Consider your own safety; do not attempt to capture or kill the snake.

2. Call EMS.

3. Keep the victim as still as possible with the bitten area below the level of the heart.

4. Wash the bite with running water if available and apply a sterile bandage over the bite.

5. If available, use an elastic bandage to lightly compress the tissues above the snakebite, working your way up the affected limb. Do not apply the bandage so tightly as to cut off blood flow. You should be able to fit two fingers underneath the bandage.

6. Make note of a description of the snake and hand over this information to EMS.

7. Provide reassurance and monitor vital signs.

Common Snakebite First Aid Myths

There are a number of myths regarding the correct first aid treatment for a snakebite. Unfortunately, these myths could make the situation worse and cause the victim further harm. Do *not*:

- Apply a tight tourniquet to cut off blood supply.
- Cut or bite into the wound to remove the snake venom.
- Attempt to suck out the snake venom.
- Give the victim any alcohol or caffeine to drink.

These treatments are no longer recommended and may cause the victim more harm than good.

Insect Stings

Many insects have the ability to bite and sting. Wasp stings are the most common type of insect sting, as wasps can be aggressive and sting without much provocation. Bees and certain types of ants can also bite and sting. The majority of insect stings cause a local reaction around the sting site. Often the area is painful, red, and swollen but improves after several days. Some people may develop a serious life-threatening allergic reaction to insect stings; this is known as anaphylaxis and can be fatal within minutes if left untreated. (See Chapter 7 for more information on how to recognize and treat a victim with suspected anaphylaxis.)

Most minor insect stings will heal within a couple of days. In some cases the sting site may become infected and require treatment with antibiotics. Be vigilant for the signs of infection (see sidebar, Watch Out for Infection) and seek medical advice if concerned.

First Aid Treatment for an Insect Sting

1. Look for an embedded stinger in the wound. If you can see a stinger, attempt to carefully remove it by brushing it away along the same angle as it entered the skin. Try to avoid using tweezers, as this can compress the stinger and squeeze more venom into the wound.

2. Clean the area with running water to reduce the risk of infection.

3. Elevate the area if a limb is affected and apply ice to reduce the swelling.

4. Medication such as antihistamines can reduce the itching from an insect sting.

5. Monitor the area for signs of infection developing (see sidebar, Watch Out for Infection).

6. Call EMS if the victim becomes unwell or displays any signs of developing a serious allergic reaction.

Watch Out for Infection

Insect stings are at risk of becoming infected. Watch out for these warning signs that may indicate an infected insect bite:

- Increasing pain
- A rapidly spreading red area around the wound
- Swelling

- Pus discharging from the wound
- High temperature (fever)
- Swollen glands near the wound

Do not delay seeking medical attention if you are concerned an insect bite is infected. If left untreated, the infection could spread to the bloodstream and cause blood poisoning (septicemia).

Tick Bite

Ticks are small parasites that feed on the blood of animals and humans. They are found in most countries but are especially common in warmer climates. Since ticks feed on blood, they can spread serious diseases such as Lyme disease and tick-borne encephalitis. Lyme disease is the most common infection spread by ticks and is becoming more common in North America. Approximately 300,000 Americans are affected by Lyme disease each year, and this number is increasing. The northeastern United States reports the most cases of Lyme disease, as this area has the highest population of ticks. You can reduce the risk of tick-borne diseases by taking steps to prevent being bitten. Try to wear long sleeve tops and long trousers when walking in tick-prone areas. In addition, you can repel ticks by using commercially available repellent sprays. If you find a tick, it should be removed as soon as possible; the longer the tick stays attached to you, the greater the risk of it passing on diseases.

Medical Terminology

Lyme disease is also known as *Lyme borreliosis*.

First Aid Treatment for a Tick Bite

1. Remove the tick as soon as possible using tweezers or a specialized tick remover; grasp the tick at the head end close to the skin and gently remove, using firm pressure.

2. Clean the bite with running water if available and cover with a sterile dressing.

3. Seek medical advice; the victim may require antibiotics to prevent Lyme disease.

4. If medical help is delayed, monitor the victim for the signs and symptoms of Lyme disease (see sidebar, Signs and Symptoms of Lyme Disease).

Signs and Symptoms of Lyme Disease

- A circular red rash around the bite known as a target lesion or bull's-eye rash that persists for several weeks
- Muscle ache

- Headache
- High temperature (fever)
- Swollen glands
- Lethargy and fatigue

Don't Use Matchsticks

Using a matchstick to burn a tick is not recommended as a way of removing the tick from the skin. In some cases, burning the tick can worsen the bite and increase the risk of infection by causing the tick to regurgitate its contents into the victim.

Jellyfish Stings

Stings from jellyfish are always a risk when in the open water. There are many varieties of jellyfish, and they range from completely harmless to potentially deadly. The box jellyfish is considered one of the most dangerous sea creatures in the world, though luckily these jellyfish are very rare in the waters around the United States. You can take steps to protect yourself from jellyfish stings by wearing a protective wetsuit and following local warning signs. Lifeguards may close beaches and swimming areas to protect people when a large swarm of jellyfish appears.

Jellyfish stings can be intensely painful, and the first aid treatment focuses on breaking down the jellyfish venom to reduce the pain and inflammation. You also need to be vigilant for signs of a severe reaction to the sting. Although it's a rare possibility, jellyfish stings can be rapidly fatal, especially when the victim has an allergy to jellyfish venom. If the victim shows signs of a severe reaction, you'll need to act quickly to summon emergency medical help and be prepared to perform cardiopulmonary resuscitation (CPR) if she or he stops breathing (see Cardiopulmonary Resuscitation (CPR) in Chapter 3).

Signs and Symptoms of a Jellyfish Sting

Signs of a jellyfish sting causing local irritation include:

- Pain
- Swelling
- Red marks on the skin
- Jellyfish tentacles stuck to the skin

Signs of a major reaction to a jellyfish sting include:

- Difficulty in breathing
- Reduced level of consciousness
- Seizures
- Vomiting

First Aid Treatment for a Jellyfish Sting

1. Remove the victim from the water as soon as possible while considering your own safety.

2. Call EMS or seek assistance from lifeguards if the victim displays any signs of a severe reaction or you are concerned that the victim is deteriorating.

3. Wear gloves and use tweezers to remove any tentacles still stuck to the skin.

4. Wash the area with vinegar as soon as possible. There is some evidence that vinegar will deactivate the stinging cells of the jellyfish. If vinegar is not available, use seawater, although it is much less effective.

5. Bathe the area in hot water (as hot as tolerated) for at least ten to twenty minutes or until the pain has subsided. Be careful not to cause burns to the victim.

6. Seek medical advice if the symptoms do not improve or the pain is not controllable with simple painkillers.

Don't Use Urine

Urinating on a jellyfish sting is a common first aid myth. There is no evidence that urine helps with the pain or swelling from a jellyfish sting. In fact, in some cases the urine may react with the jellyfish cells and worsen the symptoms from a sting.

Appendix A
FIRST AID TECHNIQUES

Effective Handwashing to Protect Yourself from Infection

Performing proper handwashing is one of the most effective ways to stop the spread of contagious diseases such as the common cold, influenza, and stomach viruses. You should aim to perform handwashing at regular intervals to reduce the risk of infection to yourself and the victim. For handwashing to be effective, it needs to be performed thoroughly. Let's take a look at how to properly clean your hands.

First, the most effective way to wash your hands is with running water and soap. Hand sanitizer gels are less effective, especially if your hands are visibly dirty. However, if you have no access to running water, then using hand sanitizer gel is much better than not cleaning your hands at all. The Centers for Disease Control and Prevention (CDC) recommend using an alcohol hand sanitizer gel with minimum concentration of 60 percent alcohol to provide effective protection against germs.

Effective handwashing should take at least forty seconds to a minute, with the scrubbing part taking a minimum of twenty seconds to complete. This time is required to effectively remove all the germs and dirt from your hands. Quickly rinsing your hands underneath a tap is unlikely to remove germs from your hands and will not protect you from catching or passing on a dangerous infection. So don't rush handwashing!

How to Perform Effective Handwashing

1. Turn on the tap and adjust the water to a warm, comfortable temperature; wet your hands and apply soap.

2. Rub the palms of your hands together to lather the soap.

3. Place your right hand over the back of your left hand then swap to clean the backs of your hands.

4. Rub palm to palm with interlocked fingers and clean the backs of the fingers.

5. Grasp the left thumb with the opposite hand, use a rotational scrub to clean the thumb, and then swap and clean the right thumb.

6. Clean the tips of the fingers by scrubbing them against the palm of the opposite hand; make sure to pay attention to the fingernails.

7. Finally, scrub down to both wrists—a commonly forgotten area.

8. Rinse both hands thoroughly with running water and use your elbow, or a hand towel, to turn the tap off.

9. Dry your hands using a disposable towel (see sidebar, Towels Carry Germs).

Towels Carry Germs

Believe it or not, reusable towels in our homes can easily become contaminated with dangerous bacteria. Damp towels are a perfect breeding ground for germs and research has shown these towels are often responsible for transmitting germs and infection. Disposable hand towels should ideally be used whenever you are washing your hands to reduce the risk of your clean hands becoming contaminated.

Applying a Pressure Bandage to Stop Bleeding

A pressure bandage is used to cover a major wound and stop bleeding. The bandage has two parts. First, a sterile pad, which is placed over the wound to cover it. Second, the elastic tail of the bandage attached to the sterile pad, which is used to wrap around the injury and apply pressure over the wound. All first aid kits should contain pressure bandages to enable you to treat wounds effectively. Because pressure bandages are sterile (free from germs), they will have an expiration date printed on the package. After this date, the bandage may no longer be completely sterile and could introduce infection into the wound.

How to Apply a Pressure Bandage

1. Choose a pressure bandage large enough to cover the entire wound; check that the bandage is up to date.

2. Ensure you are wearing disposable gloves to protect you from the victim's blood.

3. Open the sterile packaging of the bandage, taking care not to touch the sterile pad, as this could risk introducing infection.

4. Place the sterile pad directly over the wound and apply firm pressure.

5. Wrap the long tail of the bandage firmly around the sterile pad to keep pressure applied over the wound.

6. Continue wrapping the long tail around the sterile pad, ensuring the edges of the pad are covered.

7. Tie the two ends of the bandage directly over the wound.

The Complete First Aid Pocket Guide

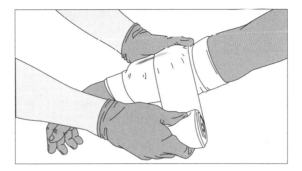

Applying a pressure bandage to stop bleeding from a wound and prevent infection.

Making a Sling for a Broken Arm

Most first aid kits contain triangular-shaped bandages to make arm slings. If an arm is broken, a sling can help by reducing movement until the victim can seek medical assistance.

How to Make a Sling

1. Place the triangular bandage underneath the injured arm with the middle point of the triangle sitting beneath the victim's elbow (think "point to the joint" to remember this).

2. Place the top end of the triangular bandage over the victim's opposite shoulder.

3. Bring the bottom end of the sling up and over the forearm and tie to the side of the victim's neck.

4. Ensure the sling is fully supporting the elbow and wrist.

5. Secure the point of the triangle with tape or a safety pin. In the event a triangular bandage is not available, you can improvise a sling with a scarf or a coat. As long as the arm is supported, it doesn't matter what material is used to make the sling.

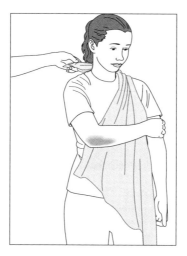

Arm sling, steps 1 and 2.

The Complete First Aid Pocket Guide

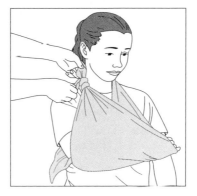

Arm sling, steps 3 and 4.

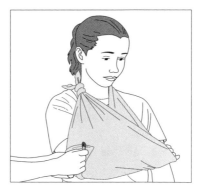

Arm sling, step 5.

Strapping a Sprained Ankle to Provide Support

Sprains and strains to the ankle can be managed by using the PRICE first aid treatment (see Chapter 4). Bandaging an injured ankle can provide support to the joint and reduce inflammation and swelling. Most first aid kits contain elastic bandages for use in this situation. You can also buy specialized ankle supports; however, these are not normally available in most first aid kits. If you are going to strap a sprained ankle, you need to be careful not to apply the bandage so tightly as to constrict blood supply to the foot. The bandage should provide comfortable support to the joint but not be so tight as to cut off blood flow to the area beyond the bandage.

There are many different methods to strap an ankle. The following is one of the most common methods used.

How to Strap an Ankle

1. Open up the elastic bandage.
2. Start at the toes, where they join the rest of the foot; tips of the toes are left unwrapped.
3. Start bandaging the foot by wrapping the bandage several times around the body of the foot.
4. Each new wrap of the bandage should overlap the previous wrap by approximately half as you work your way up the foot.

5. At the ankle, wrap the bandage in a figure-eight around the back of the ankle.

6. After strapping the ankle itself, work up the calf as far as the bandage will reach to provide additional support.

7. The bandage needs to be applied firmly to provide support but shouldn't be so tight as to constrict blood flow to the limb.

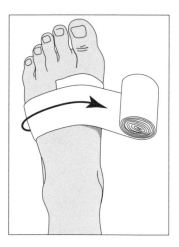

Starting where the toes join the rest of the foot, bandage the foot by wrapping the bandage several times around the body of the foot. Each new wrap of the bandage should overlap the previous wrap by approximately half as you work your way up the foot.

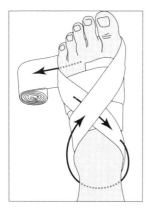

At the ankle, wrap the bandage in a figure-eight motion around the back of the ankle.

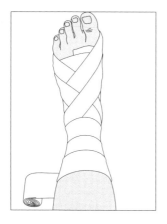

After strapping the ankle itself, work up the calf as far as the bandage will reach to provide additional support.

Seek Medical Attention If You Suspect a Fracture

Telling the difference between a badly sprained ankle and a fractured one is very difficult, even for a medical professional! Often, an X-ray is required to check for a fracture in the ankle. Always seek medical attention if you are concerned that the victim may have fractured her ankle.

Irrigating an Eye to Remove a Foreign Body

You'll need to act quickly if a victim has sustained a foreign body in his eye. Irrigation can remove the object if it is superficial. Never attempt to remove an object that is embedded in the eye. (See Chapter 4 for more information on treating a victim with a foreign body in his eye.) You'll always need to seek professional advice from a doctor or eye specialist to ensure no permanent damage has been caused to the eye. The tissues of the eye are very delicate, and even a small foreign body, such as a piece of grit or metal, can scratch the surface of the eye.

How to Irrigate an Eye

1. Sit the victim down.

2. Wash your hands with soap and running water.

3. Put on disposable gloves.

4. Inspect the eye to find the foreign object. Only attempt to remove superficial small objects with irrigation.

5. Tilt the head backward and to the side of the affected eye; place a towel (if available) to cover the victim's clothing on the affected side.

6. Pour clean water or sterile eyewash solution into the inner corner of his eye; you are aiming to wash away the object from the surface of the eye.

7. Reinspect the eye to see if the object has been removed.

8. Seek professional medical advice.

Bandaging a Blister

Blisters can be bandaged to protect the area from further damage and to reduce the risk of infection. Remember, it is not advised to burst blisters since this can increase the risk of infection. (See Chapter 4 for more information on the correct first aid for a victim with a blister.)

How to Bandage a Blister

1. Wash your hands with soap and running water.
2. Apply disposable gloves.
3. If the blister is small, apply a regular bandage or specialized blister bandage to cover the area; make sure to check that the padded area of the bandage is large enough to cover the entire blister without any of the adhesive material sticking to the blister.
4. If the blister is large, cover with a piece of gauze and secure in place loosely with a bandage.

Appendix B
FIRST AID KIT LISTS

Home First Aid Kit

- Disposable apron and eye protection
- Disposable gloves (assorted sizes)
- Elastic bandages
- First aid guide (such as *The Complete First Aid Pocket Guide*)
- Flashlight
- Foil blanket
- Hypoallergenic tape
- Large aspirin tablet
- List of your prescribed medications
- Local emergency contact details
- Notepad and pen
- Resuscitation face shield
- Safety pins
- Scissors

- Sterile eyewash solution
- Sterile gauze swabs
- Sterile tweezers
- Sterile wound dressings (assorted sizes)
- Topical antibiotic cream/ointment
- Triangular bandages
- Waterproof bandages (assorted sizes)

Vehicle First Aid Kit

- Blanket
- Bottled water
- Disposable apron and eye protection
- Disposable gloves (assorted sizes)
- Elastic bandages
- Emergency warning triangle
- First aid guide (such as *The Complete First Aid Pocket Guide*)
- Flashlight
- Foil blanket
- High-visibility jacket
- Hypoallergenic tape
- List of your prescribed medications
- Local emergency contact details

- Notepad and pen
- Resuscitation face shield
- Safety pins
- Scissors
- Sterile eyewash solution
- Sterile gauze swabs
- Sterile tweezers
- Sterile wound dressings (assorted sizes)
- Triangular bandages
- Waterproof bandages (assorted sizes)

Outdoor First Aid Kit
- Blister bandages (assorted sizes)
- Compass and map
- Disposable gloves (assorted sizes)
- Elastic bandages
- Emergency shelter/survival blanket
- First aid guide (such as *The Complete First Aid Pocket Guide*)
- Flashlight
- Foil blanket
- High-energy food snacks (e.g., chocolate bar)
- Hypoallergenic tape

- Large aspirin tablet
- List of your prescribed medications
- Local emergency contact details
- Notepad and pen
- Resuscitation face shield
- Safety pins
- Scissors
- Sterile gauze swabs
- Sterile tweezers
- Sterile wound dressings (assorted sizes)
- Topical antibiotic cream
- Triangular bandages
- Waterproof bandages (assorted sizes)

The Overall Aims of First Aid

- **P**reserve the life of the victim
- **P**revent worsening of the situation
- **P**romote recovery from the injury or illness

Gathering Important Information from a Victim: AMPLE History

- **A**llergies: Do you have any known allergies to medication or food? Do you carry an EpiPen?
- **M**edication: What medication do you take from your doctor? Do you take any additional medication that you buy from a store?
- **P**ast medical history: Do you have any medical conditions? Have you had any recent surgery?

- Last oral intake (food or fluid): When was the last time you had anything to eat or drink?
- Events leading up to the incident: What happened prior to the incident or you becoming unwell?

Assessment of an Unresponsive Victim: DR ABC Action Plan
- **D**anger
- **R**esponse
- **A**irway
- **B**reathing
- **C**PR (if required)

Cardiopulmonary Resuscitation: CAB
- Compressions
- Airway
- Breathing

Signs of a Stroke (Brain Attack): FAST
- **F**acial droop
- **A**rm weakness
- **S**lurred speech
- **T**ime to call EMS

Signs and Symptoms of a Fracture: PLASTIC

- **P**ain
- **L**oss of movement
- **A**ngulation of the limb
- **S**welling
- **T**enderness
- **I**rregularity
- **C**repitus (a cracking or grating sound)

Treatment of a Soft-Tissue Injury: PRICE

1. **P**rotect the area from further injury
2. **R**est the injury
3. **I**ce the injury to reduce swelling
4. **C**ompress the injury gently with a bandage or support
5. **E**levate the limb to reduce swelling and pain

Appendix D
A-TO-Z LIST OF AILMENTS AND CONDITIONS

Amputation

Anaphylaxis (severe allergic reaction)

Animal bites

Asthma

Black eye

Blisters

Broken nose

Bronchiolitis

Chemical burns

Chicken pox

Choking (adult)

Choking (child or baby)

Common cold

Croup

Crush injuries

Dehydration

Diabetic hyperglycemia (high blood sugar)

Diabetic hypoglycemia (low blood sugar)

Diarrhea

Dislocations

Earache

Emergency childbirth

Fainting

Febrile seizures

Foreign body in eye

Foreign object lodged in ear

Foreign object lodged in nose

Fractures (closed)

Fractures (open)

Frostbite

Head injuries

Headache

Heart attack

Heatstroke

Hyperventilation (panic attacks)

Hypothermia

Influenza

Insect stings

Jellyfish stings

Knocked-out teeth

Lightning strike

Major burns

Meningitis

Minor burns

Minor wounds (cuts and grazes)

Motion sickness

Nausea and vomiting

Near drowning

Neck and back injuries

Nosebleeds

Poison ivy, oak, and sumac

Poisoning

Puncture wounds

Seizures

Severe bleeding

Shock

Snake bites

Soft-tissue injuries (sprains and strains)

Splinters

Stroke (brain attack)

Sunburn

Tick bites

Unresponsive adult

Unresponsive baby or child

Index

The Complete First Aid Pocket Guide

About the Author

JOHN FURST is an experienced emergency medical technician and qualified first aid and CPR instructor. His instructor career began with the Red Cross, and he now works as a freelance first aid instructor and assessor. He has worked as an EMT and first responder for many years and is able to draw upon his extensive real-world experience when teaching first aid classes. John is passionate about first aid and believes everyone should have the skills and confidence to take action in an emergency situation. John runs the popular first aid blog FirstAidforFree.com, where he regularly writes about current first aid topics and the latest best practices.